THE ULTIMATE

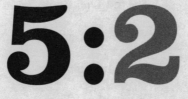

DIET
RECIPE BOOK

The only 5:2 recipe book you will ever need

THE ULTIMATE

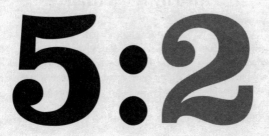

5:2

DIET
RECIPE BOOK

Easy, Calorie Counted Fast Day Meals You'll Love

KATE HARRISON

This edition first published in Great Britain in 2013 by
Orion
an imprint of the Orion Publishing Group Ltd
Orion House, 5 Upper St Martin's Lane,
London WC2H 9EA
An Hachette UK Company

A CIP catalogue record for this book is available from the British Library.

Printed in Great Britain by CPI Group (UK) Ltd, Croydon, CR0 4YY
Photographer: Andrew Hayes-Watkins
Food consultants and stylists: Anna Burges-Lumsden and Lisa Harrison
Prop stylist: Guiliana Casarotti

The Orion Publishing Group's policy is to use papers that are natural, renewable and recyclable
and made from wood grown in sustainable forests. The logging and manufacturing processes are
expected to conform to the environmental regulations of the country of origin.

Every effort has been made to ensure that the information
in the book is accurate. The information in this book will be relevant to the majority of people
but may not be applicable in each individual case so it is advised that professional medical
advice is obtained for specific health matters. Neither the publisher nor author accepts any
legal responsibility for any personal injury or other damage or loss arising from the use of
the information in this book. Anyone making a change in their diet should consult their GP
especially if pregnant, infirm, elderly or under 16.

Every effort has been made to fulfil requirements with regard to reproducing
copyright material. The author and publisher will be glad to rectify any omissions
at the earliest opportunity.

www.orionbooks.co.uk

Contents

WELCOME TO 5:2: The Delicious, Flexible, Guilt-Free Approach to Healthy Eating   **1**

Introduction   3

How This Book Works   7

Important Safety Note   8

PART ONE: HOW TO 5:2   **9**

PART TWO: 5:2 FOOD   **33**

1: Great Starts

Anytime Breakfasts and Brunches   41

5:2 Know-How: The Store Cupboard   61

2: Super Soups

To Keep You Full on Fast Days   68

5:2 Know-How: Tools of the Trade   95

3: Hot Stuff

To Spice Up Fast Days   100

5:2 Know-How: Fast Day Flavours   127

4: Comfort Food

Big-Hearted Dishes for Flatter Bellies   132

5:2 Know-How: Family Eating   161

5: Salad Days

Hot and Cold Salads for Every Season   164

5:2 Know-How: Veg Box Magic   202

6: 5:2 To Go

Packed Lunches (and picnics!)   206

5:2 Know-How: Fasting on a Budget   230

7: 5:2 On Tour

A Taste of Holidays Around the Globe   232

5:2 Know-How: Holidays and Celebrations   264

8: 5:2 Treats

Delicious Desserts and Drinks   266

5:2 Know-How: 5:2 for Life   295

9: 5:2 Extras

Sauces, Dressings and Swaps   297

5:2 Know-How: 5:2 Final Inspirations   324

10: 5:2 Menu Plans Made Easy

Four Weeks of Fasting Meal Planning   326

PART THREE: 5:2 TOOL KIT   **333**

Recipes Listed by Calorie Count Per Serving   333

Calorie Counter   338

Glossary   349

BMI Chart   351

Online Links and Further Reading   352

Acknowledgements   354

Index   356

Recipe Index   357

WELCOME TO

5:2

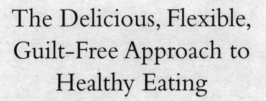

The Delicious, Flexible,
Guilt-Free Approach to
Healthy Eating

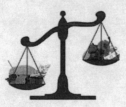

May 2013

Dear Reader,

Do you want to eat the foods you love and rediscover your appetite for fresh, delicious meals? Would you like to improve your health and lose weight as well as any guilt you feel about eating? **You're in the right place . . .**

I admit it sounds too good to be true. But if you're already following 5:2, you know this approach really works. It's simple, it costs nothing, and it's changing lives.

In this book, I hope to inspire you to eat even better and tastier food. The dishes and ideas make me happy – and they make following 5:2 easier and healthier than before. This is the opposite of dull 'diet' food that makes you feel you're being punished for something!

If you're new to 5:2 and are struggling to believe a 'diet' could be so easy, I know where you're coming from. I'm a natural sceptic, especially when it comes to weight-loss crazes that promise the earth and fail to deliver. I've tried most of them over the years, and ended up bigger than ever. Until now.

From sceptic to 5:2 fan . . .

This has been the easiest eating plan I've ever followed. In nine months I've lost 11kg (25lb), which is more than 15 per cent of my original weight. I've dropped almost three dress sizes and my size is no longer putting my health in danger. Plus, research suggests that the 5:2 diet reduces my risk of developing cancer, heart disease, type 2 diabetes and Alzheimer's disease.

3

As important, for me, is how my attitude to food has changed for the better. I've always loved cooking and eating out, but all the guilt and emotional baggage has gone.

My friends tell me I sound a bit like I've joined a cult, but they also tell me how much better I look. And this cult has no weird supplements, revolting food-replacement shakes or bizarre rituals. It's just the simplest, cheapest approach to healthy eating around. And as you read this book, you'll discover the stories of men and women of all ages and backgrounds who are making 5:2 work for them too. So what is it that so many people love about the 5:2 diet?

5:2 means great food

5:2 is all about fabulous food: variety, freshness and taste.

FIVE days a week, you'll eat without restriction – though after fasting you'll probably find you eat less because it takes less to satisfy your newly heightened sense of taste and smell.

TWO days a week you'll eat less than you usually do, but from an almost endless selection of great food. The list includes dishes like Portobello Mushroom Rarebit, Thai Curry, Pizza, Skinny Chilli con Carne, Skinny Chicken Kievs, Sweet Potato Falafels, Lemon and Pork Meatballs and even a Jaffa Cake Chocolate Mousse! Proof that you don't have to sacrifice flavour on your Fast Days.

5:2 means freedom

5:2 liberates you from calorie counting day after monotonous day. It helps you to understand what 'fuel' your body really needs to function, and it frees you to enjoy a lovingly prepared family meal or a really tasty cooked breakfast without the guilt.

5:2 means good health

This approach helps you lose weight, which will improve your overall health. But the Fast Days also help your body repair itself, making sure your cells and systems are working as efficiently as possible. The benefits include mental sharpness, a better response to insulin and a lowered risk of a range of disabling and life-shortening conditions.

This book is about easy, delicious meals to savour

The *Ultimate 5:2 Diet Recipe Book* is a hands-on guide to creating dishes with maximum flavour but minimum calories for Fast Days. In addition, it offers advice on how to eat the rest of the time, and provides all the essential information you need to start 5:2 tomorrow – or even today, if you're reading this before breakfast!

Pre-prepared foods can be convenient, but since starting 5:2 I've wanted to cook fresher food for my partner and myself. I can't afford to spend hours shopping or cooking each day, so I've developed time-saving recipes and techniques that mean I know exactly what's gone into my dishes without having to slave away for hours.

This book is about community

The questions, tips and food passions of our brilliant 5:2 dieters on Facebook www.facebook.com/groups/the52diet and the 5:2 website www.the5-2dietbook.com have influenced every aspect of this book.

The Facebook group started in September 2012 when I invited a few friends to share experiences of fasting. I'd just watched the BBC Horizon programme *Eat, Fast and Live Longer* with Dr Michael Mosley; with diabetes and breast cancer running in my family, I decided to try the fasting approach for the health benefits as much as the (much-needed!) weight loss.

The only frustration was that I couldn't find a practical guidebook, so I thought the group would help us share recipes and ideas. As numbers grew, and I became more and more absorbed in researching the science as well as the practicalities, I realised I could write the book I couldn't find, incorporating the experiences of the people who were fasting alongside me.

The 5:2 Diet Book was published in November 2012, and that tiny group of friends has now grown to a lively forum of more than 5,000 people. They've been asking for a follow-up book, with recipes and menus featuring their favourite ingredients and cuisines: from cheese feasts to sweet treats, veggie dishes to meaty stews, Italian pasta dishes to Indian curries. They're all in here.

And do you want to know the best thing of all? Despite months of intensive recipe writing and testing, I've continued to lose weight and have now reached my goal... The proof of the pudding (and starter and main course) really *is* in the eating.

Happy fasting – and feasting,
Kate

How This Book Works

PART 1

How to 5:2 introduces the approach with a summary of the health benefits and answers to the questions I'm asked most often, including: What should I eat on Fast Days? Can I really eat what I like on Feast Days without calorie counting? How does exercise fit into 5:2?

PART 2

5:2 Food is the main event. This part is packed with recipes and inspiration; from super soups to salads, comfort food and world cuisine, there are ideas to suit you. There is also extra information to inspire and help make the diet work for you.

5:2 Lives shares real-life examples of how 5:2 works for people with different lifestyles and needs. Read very honest food diaries, success stories and tips, plus a featured recipe from each of our contributing dieters.

5:2 Know-How reveals the ideas, techniques and ingredients that will help make your Fast Days a breeze. These sections cover all aspects of the diet from 5:2 on a budget to the store-cupboard supplies you'll need to keep you on track.

5:2 Meal Plans – four weeks' worth of meal planning for your Fast Days with ideas to suit your needs, whether you want breakfast, lunch and supper, or a grand three-course dinner with friends.

PART 3
The 5:2 Tool Kit includes a customised calorie counter, links to research and web resources, plus a handy reference listing all the dishes in the book according to their calorie count.

Time to get cooking . . . Whether you're brand new to 5:2, or you're looking for inspiration to make your Fast Days even better, it's time to dive into food, glorious food . . . *bon appétit!*

Important Safety Note

You should always consult a doctor before making any new dietary changes.

This book is written for information only and is not intended as medical advice, or as a substitute for medical advice, diagnosis or treatment.

Children, teenagers and pregnant and breast-feeding women shouldn't fast.

If you have a chronic condition, diabetes, or any history of eating disorders, it's particularly important that you consult your doctor, specialist or diabetes nurse, before embarking on the 5:2 diet.

Finally, never disregard professional medical advice or delay starting medical treatment because of something you have read in this book.

1

HOW TO

5:2

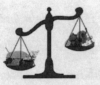

What is 5:2?

What makes 5:2 different?

*Should I do my Fast Days one after the other,
or more than two per week?*

How many calories should I consume on Fast Days?

How do I calculate my personal Fast Day calorie limit?

When should I eat on Fast Days?

What can I eat on Fast Days?

How will I feel on a Fast Day?

What about hunger?

Can I exercise when I fast?

What about the other five Feast Days?
Should I calorie count?

Do I need to worry about starvation mode?

I've heard of half-fasts, 18:6 or eight-hour windows.
Should I be trying these too?

How much weight should I aim to lose?

How much weight will I lose?

How can I keep track of my 5:2 progress?

What if my weight loss stalls?

How does 5:2 affect the body?

What about 5:2 and the mind?

How long can I stay on 5:2?

Where can I get more support?

A word about words

What is 5:2?

THE SIMPLEST, HEALTHIEST, CHEAPEST DIET YOU'LL EVER TRY

5:2 is a flexible approach to healthy eating that involves cutting your calorie consumption to 25 per cent of your energy needs on two days each week, and eating normally for the other five days. And that's it!

The simplicity of this diet is what makes it so irresistible to many of us. You either do some basic maths to work out your calorie 'limit' or opt for a goal based on average energy needs: 500 for women and 600 for men (see page 14). We call the limited days 'Fast Days', even though you do get to eat tempting and filling meals. I call the other five days my 'Feast Days' because all food feels like a feast on those days, but you'll find that some people use the term 'Feed', 'Free' or even simply 'Normal' Days.

You can even fine-tune the number of days you fast, depending on how quickly you want to lose weight – so a 4:3 approach means three Fast Days, which should increase the speed of weight loss. Or 6:1 is the choice for many who've either

11

reached their target weight, or are following this lifestyle for the great health benefits. More on the science on pages 28–29!

If you stick to the two days at the 500–600 calories guideline, you'll begin to reap the benefits. But if you're anything like me, you'll want to know more about why you should try this diet, why it's different and what it'll do for your weight and your general health.

So here I'll answer all the questions I had when I started out, as well as the questions that crop up again and again on our forums. But feel free to go straight to the recipes, if you're in the mood for food.

I've tried loads of diets and always put the weight back on, what makes 5:2 different?

All weight-loss diets rely on you consuming less energy (food, measured in calories) than you use up in your daily life. The trouble with measuring – or counting – calories is that it's boring and labour-intensive, and it can make you obsessed with food.

On one level, 5:2 is just a different way to manage eating less. It's less monotonous because you only have to count for two days a week: the ultimate part-time diet. On the other days you can still celebrate family occasions, go for drinks and a meal with friends and enjoy the foods you love.

That flexibility makes it *so* much more likely that you'll stick to it long term. And weight loss isn't the whole story; 5:2 is also different because of the potential health benefits, which are very motivating.

Should I do my Fast Days one after the other, and can I do more than two?

It's easier and more manageable to separate your Fast Days – for example, doing Monday and Wednesday or Tuesday and Thursday. That's particularly true while you're getting used to the Fast Days. It's so much easier to stick to your limit when you know that tomorrow you can eat what you like.

Once you're used to fasting, you can choose to do the two days together. I do that occasionally, when it suits my schedule. I find it a little tougher than one day but it's still easier than full-time dieting.

You also don't have to do the same days each week; you can fit them around work commitments or family occasions. Planning the best days to do your fast is one of the keys to overall success.

You can do more than two days, and many people on our forums switch between 5:2 and 4:3, where they do three Fast Days. It increases the calorie deficit (the difference between what you eat and the energy you need), which will usually mean you'll lose weight faster. Another variation is Alternate Day Fasting (ADF), where you fast every other day.

It's up to you, though I advise against doing more than two Fast Days together because it may trigger some unhelpful changes in how your body is using energy.

Finally, if you don't have weight to lose or have reached your goal weight, then 6:1, fasting just once a week, is a good option if you want the health benefits this plan offers.

How many calories should I consume on Fast Days?

We're aiming for around one quarter of what our bodies use up on a typical day: that figure is known as Daily Calorie Requirement (DCR) or Total Daily Energy Expenditure (TDEE).

There are two ways to set your limit: one is to work on the average requirements for men and women, and the other is to do personal calculations.

For most of us, the averages work just fine. Most moderately active women use around 1,800–2,000 calories per day: a quarter of the upper figure gives us a Fast Day calorie limit of 500. Moderately active men need on average 2,400 calories a day, so they get an extra 100 calories per Fast Day, meaning a total Fast Day calorie limit of 600 calories.

It may be worth calculating your own limits if you are much smaller, taller, heavier, lighter or more or less active than the average person. A smaller woman who does no exercise will need significantly fewer calories than a taller, overweight woman who is training for a marathon. The larger we are – and therefore the more weight we are carrying – the more calories we need to sustain our current size. It is, incidentally, one of the reasons why weight loss on traditional diets can be harder to sustain as the slimmer we are, the fewer calories we need. However, if we switch to 6:1 (one Fast Day per week) after reaching our goal weight, it helps us stay aware of what our appetite is telling us we really need.

How do I calculate my personal Fast Day calorie limit?

The easiest way to do this is using an online calculator to work out your calorie requirements/energy expenditure (DCR/TDEE). There are links to these in the resources section (see pages 352–353). You then divide that total by four, and that's your calorie limit for your Fast Days.

The formula for working out your energy needs takes into account your gender, age, current weight, height and also your current levels of physical activity, but it's really important to understand that all of these are based on *estimates*. Discovering exactly how many calories you burn is an expensive and time-consuming process. Different online calculators may give slightly different results; don't get too hung up on a difference of a few calories.

The other thing to know is that there are two main formulas used to calculate the DCR/TDEE: the Harris Benedict and the Mifflin St Jeor. Most online calculators use the former, but the latter is actually said to be more accurate.

If you want to do it yourself, you'll need to first calculate your Basal Metabolic Rate (BMR), which is the number of calories you need to keep your basic functions going without losing weight.

I'm going to use the Mifflin St Jeor formula, but remember that if you get different results from an online calculator, they're probably using Harris Benedict.

Mifflin St Jeor BMR Formula

Male: (10 × weight in kg) + (6.25 × height in cm) − (5 × your age) + 5
= BMR

Female: (10 × weight in kg) + (6.25 × height in cm) − (5 × your age) − 161
= BMR

I'll give my numbers as an example. After losing 11kg (25 lbs) on this diet, I now weigh 61.7kg (136 lbs). My height is 163cm (5ft 4in) and I am 45.

617 (10 x 61.7) + 1,019 (6.25 x 163) − 225 (5 x 45) − 161
= BMR of 1,250

Please keep in mind that this is your BMR: it's enough to keep you going, but it's not what you use to calculate your Fast Day calorie limit. For this, we need to factor in how active you are to determine your total Daily Calorie Requirement (DCR) or Total Daily Energy Expenditure (TDEE). We do that by multiplying your BMR by a figure depending on how much exercise you do or how active your job is.

Little or no exercise: BMR x 1.2
Light exercise (1−3 days per week): BMR x 1.375
Moderate exercise (3−5 days per week): BMR x 1.55
Very active (6−7 days per week): BMR x 1.725
Extra active (very active and physical job): BMR x 1.9

So in my case, I currently do light exercise (busy writing this book!), which means my DCR/TDEE is:

1,250 (BMR) x 1.375 = **1,719**

So if I consume roughly 1,700 calories each day, my weight should stay stable.

The final sum for calculating your Fast Day limit is to divide your DCR/TDEE by four. In my case this equals 430 calories. This is lower than the average because I am slightly shorter than average, and I also weigh less since I started out on 5:2! I try to stick to this on my Fast Days but I suspect my weight loss would have been only a little slower had I aimed for 500 calories.

As a comparison, I did the same sums online using the Harris Benedict method and it gave me 1,832, with a Fast Day limit of 458 calories.

If you lose a lot of weight, you should recalculate your limits, as your DCR/TDEE decreases along with your weight – UNLESS you step up your activity levels, which may happen as you find you have more energy and confidence!

When should I eat on Fast Days? And how often?

You can consume your calorie allowance in one, two or even three meals, although some researchers suspect that the health benefits may be greater if you restrict yourself to just one or two meals.

You can choose to eat when it suits you, although many 5:2 dieters – me, included – have found that once they're used to Fast Days, it is easier to manage if they postpone eating until as late in the day as possible. In the past, I *always* ate breakfast, but now I find that skipping it on Fast Days means I feel less hungry during the day than when I do eat something in the morning.

You can (and should) drink plenty of water. You can also drink black coffee or tea, herb teas and diet drinks, although artificially sweetened drinks may still affect your insulin levels. If you take milk, remember to include the calories in your allowance. Some 5:2 dieters avoid milky drinks except with meals because there's evidence they can trigger the production of insulin, which may be counter-productive.

It's up to you how many meals you eat. In one major study of ADF (Alternate Daily Fasting), participants had a single meal at lunchtime on their Fast Days with good results. That makes sense to me because the body has less to 'do' in terms of digesting food, releasing insulin, etc. But if you prefer, you can eat three smaller meals, and even factor in a snack – this may be useful at first if you're worried about feeling unwell or jittery if you don't eat regularly.

The beauty of this diet compared to all the others I've tried (and abandoned) is the flexibility: you decide how to make the diet fit your life, rather than the diet dictating how to live.

On a personal note: at the start, I could never have imagined going a whole day without any food. But now I frequently eat only once or twice, so that I can eat a slightly larger meal with my partner in the evening, for example. I don't find it difficult at all.

What can I eat on Fast Days?

In theory, you can eat whatever you like – as long as you stay under your calorie limit. This book is all about making satisfying dishes that help you stay on track! In general, vegetables and small portions of lean meats, fish or eggs are more satisfying than fruit or refined carbohydrates like white bread or rice. And sweets, cakes or alcohol are best avoided as they will 'eat into' your allowance very dramatically *and* give you a sugar rush that may make you hungry again very quickly and make you less likely to succeed. There's lots of inspiration to come in the recipe and meal-planning sections later on in the book.

How will I feel on a Fast Day?

Once you're used to Fast Days, you'll almost certainly feel more energetic and positive – and you'll enjoy every mouthful of the food you prepare for yourself.

At first, though, Fast Days can take some getting used to. You may feel hungry to begin with and people sometimes report feeling the cold more or experiencing headaches; all of these are common with any new diet. Of course, if you feel very unwell, don't hesitate to stop fasting until you've seen your doctor but this is very, very unusual.

Most of us adjust very quickly to eating less on Fast Days, but it makes sense to schedule your first couple of days for when you don't have too much going on. Having said that, it's best not to clear your diary completely – most of us have found that staying busy is the best distraction from any hunger pangs.

What about hunger? Won't I be ravenous?

This is one of the biggest concerns for people new to 5:2 and yet, for most of us, the fear disappears within two or three Fast

Days. The truth is 500 or 600 calories is enough to keep you satisfied, if you choose wisely (and you're reading this book, which has lots of wise choices!).

We're so used to eating at regular times, and snacking or 'grazing' between meals, that many of us have forgotten how it feels to be hungry. At first, it can be an unsettling feeling but there are a few things to bear in mind.

First, hunger tends to come in waves and if you have a hot drink or distract yourself with a phone call, a piece of work or a quick look at the online 5:2 groups or forums, it will soon go away or diminish.

Second, this is a temporary choice you're making and one from which your body will benefit long term.

Third, getting back in touch with your appetite is one of the best things you can do in terms of developing healthier eating habits. Allowing yourself to get to the point where you are looking forward to food, where it tastes amazing and where you will know when you've had enough can be a dramatic change, and one that will benefit you all the time, not just two days a week.

Finally, remember the positive 5:2 catchphrase: *tomorrow you can eat what you like!*

Can I exercise when I fast? And can I 'buy' more calories that way?

Many of us do exercise on Fast Days and there's no medical reason why you shouldn't. It may be a good idea to wait until after your first couple of fasts before attempting it though, and to take it gently. If you feel unwell, then listen to your body and stop.

One thing to note: you shouldn't add any calories burned through exercise to your calorie allowance on a Fast Day – stick to 500–600 calories for the health benefits!

What about the five Feast Days? Should I calorie count, or can I eat whatever I like?

This is one of the most common topics in our forums and it has both a simple and a complicated answer!

The simple answer is: you can eat your favourite foods. I've done this, enjoying chocolate, cheese, treats, celebratory meals and wine, and I've lost 11kg (25 lb). I've found that removing the guilt and any restrictions has made my eating much, much more balanced overall. I don't binge on my Feast Days; everything I eat feels like a feast and I savour my food, but I stop when I'm full.

The slightly more complicated answer is that it *is* possible to 'cancel out' the calorie deficit you've created on your Fast Days if you eat an awful lot on your Feast Days. We can't change how our body uses up energy: if you eat more calories than you're burning off, you will gain weight.

However, the really interesting thing about 5:2 is the effect it has on how most of us eat. In reality, bingeing doesn't seem to happen because Fast Days have such a powerful 'reset' effect on your appetite and you quickly develop a heightened awareness of how much food your body actually needs.

Research has shown that ICR (Intermittent Calorie Restriction), doesn't lead to bingeing. In one study of people following a 4:3 plan, dieters ate between 95 per cent and 125 per cent of their DCR on the day after a Fast – so even the higher figure wasn't enough to cancel out the Fast Day deficit. In fact, most of us find we eat significantly less than before, without doing it consciously.

Many of us are happy to let this new awareness help us stay on track. Calorie counting and limited eating on Fast Days only helps us appreciate the foods we can eat on Feast days and to understand how much we really need to sate our hunger, so we naturally eat slightly less or pick healthier options.

However, a significant minority of 5:2 dieters – especially those who have been on diets for much of their adult lives – are reluctant to give up the calorie counting. If you do want to count on non-Fast Days, then your DCR/TDEE (an average of 2,000 for women, and 2,400 for men) is what you're aiming for, but your intake will vary naturally day-by-day depending on your activity levels.

The biggest concerns for me about constant calorie counting are, first, that it's boring and means that 5:2 *plus* counting is not that different from normal dieting, which could make it unsustainable. The second is that counting can become obsessive and may lead to feelings of guilt if we overdo it, which is one of the things 5:2 has freed so many people from.

If you do choose to calorie-count when you're not fasting, then our calorie-chart on pages 338–348 will come in very handy. But my advice for the long-term would be to try to relax and enjoy your food on Feast Days.

Do I need to worry about starvation mode?

No. Other low-calorie diets can trigger your body to store more fat in the long term, but not 5:2. 'Starvation mode' happens when food is perceived by the body to be scarce, but because 5:2 alternates no more than two Fast Days with normal eating, your body doesn't respond by slowing the metabolism as it might with other, more prolonged forms of calorie restriction.

I've heard of half-fasts, 18:6 or eight-hour windows. Should I be trying these too?

There are almost as many variations on 5:2 as there are people doing it, which can be confusing. No-one can agree, for example, what a 'half fast' even is! 18:6 and 8 hour 'feeding' windows involve only eating within a short 'window' during the day (6 hours out of 24, for example) and fasting the rest of the time.

After debating all the options on our forums – and seeing the confusion they can cause – I've come to the conclusion that personally, I think keeping it simple is best – one Fast Day at a time, where you consume under your limit from morning until night, and eat normally the next day

How much weight should I aim to lose?

There are several different ways to assess whether your weight could be damaging to your health. Body Mass Index (BMI) is the one most commonly used by doctors. To find out yours, use the chart in the Tool Kit (see page 351), an online calculator or the formula below.

$$BMI = \frac{\text{Weight in kg}}{(\text{Height in m}) \times (\text{Height in m})}$$

If your BMI is over 25 (or 23 for some ethnic groups) you're officially overweight. And if it's over 30, you're classed as obese. The higher the figure, the higher the statistical risk of disease.

BMI is a very general measure and it has many limitations. Another good indicator is your waist measurement, which is a strong predictor of your likelihood of developing cardiovascular disease.

'Pear-shaped' people, with larger hips and thighs, tend to have a lower risk than 'apples', who store more fat around their belly. This is because, the bigger your waist is, the higher the likelihood that you've accumulated 'visceral' fat around the vital organs. And visceral fat is associated with higher rates of Type 2 diabetes, stroke and heart disease.

The current NHS guideline is that you are at a greater risk if your waist (measured round your belly button) is more than 94cm (37 in) if you're a man and 80cm (31.5 in) if you're a woman.

Specialists now advise that we fine-tune that measurement by aiming to keep our waist measurement to less than half of our height, or a ratio of less than 0.5.

In my case, I am 163cm (5ft 4 in) tall, so my waist measurement should stay under 81.5cm (32 in). As an indicator, here's how mine has changed over time:

August 2012: Waist (81.5cm) ÷ Height (163cm) = 0.5
January 2013: Waist (75cm) ÷ Height (163cm) = 0.46
April 2013: Waist (70cm) ÷ Height (163cm) = 0.43

I know how hard it is to face the scales or use a tape measure when you feel bad about your weight, but once you begin to lose weight, you'll be glad that you were honest with yourself at the beginning because your progress will be all the more impressive.

How much weight will I lose? And how quickly?

In this book, you'll read about one couple that lost 45kg (100 lb) between them (see pages 102–105), and hear from other dieters who don't want to lose very much weight but want the health benefits that 5:2 offers.

In our forums, some people lose 2.25kg (5 lb) or more in their first week, and others never lose more than 0.2kg (0.5 lb) a week. If you're more of a tortoise than a hare, you're in good company; I was the same, but now I am very happy with my weight. In general, people with more weight to lose are likely to see more rapid losses, while that last little bit to your target is often the toughest to shift.

Dieticians estimate that to lose 0.45kg (1 lb) of weight, we need to have a 'deficit' of 3,500 calories – and to put the same amount *on,* we'd have to eat 3,500 calories more than we need.

These figures apply over any period of time. So if you're fasting for three days a week, you're likely to lose weight faster than if you're fasting for two days. I go into more detail about the numbers in *The 5:2 Diet Book*, but if you fast for two days a week, you will create a deficit of just under 3,500 calories, so you can expect to lose about a 0.45kg (1 lb) every week if you eat normally on the other days. Weight loss researchers – and dieters who've maintained their weight loss – believe that losing up to 0.45–0.8kg (1–2lb) a week is more sustainable than 'crash' dieting.

How can I keep track of my 5:2 progress?

Studies suggest that dieters who keep a record of what they eat tend to be more successful. You can either do this electronically or simply jot it down in a notebook. The brilliant thing about 5:2 is that you only need to record what you're eating on your two Fast Days.

A pocket calorie-counting book is a good option, but I find using an app or website like MyFitnessPal (www.myfitnesspal. com) makes it easy to record my calorie consumption. On the website, you can keep the information private or share it with others to help you stay motivated. You simply enter the name of the food and the quantity, and the app calculates the total number of calories (though as most of the data are provided by users, some entries may be unreliable, so be a little careful: if a count seems too good to be true, it may be inaccurate so do double-check with other sites). You can even scan the barcode of a food if you have MyFitnessPal on your phone.

Cooking from scratch involves adding up the calories for all the individual ingredients you use, but we've made it much easier in this book by giving a total calorie count per serving, plus the individual listing for each ingredient so you can adapt it to suit your tastes.

MyFitnessPal also allows you to record your weight and measurements over time.

The only thing to be wary of with MyFitnessPal is that it doesn't have a setting for 5:2, so it may tell you to eat more on a Fast Day, and if you're recording on a Feast Day too, it may tell you to eat less. The easiest way to overcome this is to set your membership to Maintain, or just ignore its advice and focus on the numbers.

What if my weight loss stalls?

Remember that your weight may fluctuate on a daily basis for many reasons. Our bodies vary day-to-day depending on what we've been eating, and for women, hormonal changes can add 2.5kg (5.5 lb) (or more) at different times of the month!

Many of the happiest 5:2 dieters on our forums only weigh themselves once a month, or not at all, instead relying on their tape measure, the fit of their clothes – and compliments – to help them monitor their progress.

If, after a couple of weeks of following the plan you're not losing weight, try adding up the calories you're eating on an average Feast Day. If it's a lot over your DCR (or the average of 2,000 for women and 2,400 for men) you could consider switching to 4:3 or Alternate Day Fasting (ADF) for a little while, or try and identify ways to cut back on Feast Day consumption without losing your pleasure in food.

Certain medical conditions can make it harder to shift

weight, so if you are confident you are following the plan correctly, it's worth discussing it with your GP.

How does 5:2 affect my health?

Weight loss is the most obvious result of 5:2, but that doesn't mean it's the most important. Your Fast Days also have an amazing effect on your body's ability to repair itself.

Research from humans and animal studies has shown that intermittent calorie restriction (the more precise term for what we call fasting) can reduce the risk of developing many cancers, cardiovascular diseases and Alzheimer's disease and other forms of dementia.

The biology is complex, but fasting triggers processes that slow down the growth of new cells, and instead boost repairs to our existing ones, to prime us for survival. One key hormone, called IGF-1, or 'insulin-like growth factor' is of particular interest. This hormone is essential for cell growth in babies and children, but in adults, raised IGF-1 is linked with biological ageing and the development of cancer. Crucially, levels of this hormone have been seen to decrease on Fast Days, which may be the key to many of the health benefits associated with intermittent calorie restriction.

But why would this be? Part of the answer may be connected to how our ancestors lived. Naturally, their lives followed a feast/fast pattern. Our bodies, therefore, evolved to take in as much energy as possible in the 'good' times, like during a harvest or when hunters brought back an animal they'd caught to eat. By 'feasting', our bodies would accumulate fat stores in reserve to keep us going during the leaner times.

It's only very recently that starvation has ceased to be a threat to most developed populations. Now, we have an incredibly wide choice of foods available to us, including all the healthy, fresh, minimally processed foods that doctors and diet experts recommend. Yet our bodies still crave the food that would have ensured the survival of our ancestors. Our bodies don't think ahead; all they can do is react to the now. So when sweet and fatty foods are on offer, we're programmed to like the taste and texture, and to eat as much as possible, so we can lay down fat stores for a nutritional 'rainy day'.

What 5:2 and fasting does is to go back to basics. I think of it as reintroducing some of the 'rainy days' our ancestors were only too familiar with, by providing less energy from food, but in a controlled way.

When we fast, our bodies respond by trying to ensure we're in the best shape for famine. That includes 'tidying up' rogue cells that are cluttering up the place, and repairing any that need help – a little like doing maintenance to get the house or car ready for a harsh winter.

When we go back to eating normally the next day, the bad times stop – but we've gained the benefits of that maintenance and housekeeping. You can read much more about these processes in *The 5:2 Diet Book,* or via the research links at the end of this book (see pages 352–353).

There's another factor, too, and that's the negative effect eating constantly has on the body. For years, we've been encouraged to snack or 'graze' between meals. However, doing this means the body is constantly digesting food and balancing out our blood sugar levels. The hormone insulin prevents levels of sugar becoming dangerously high – but it also stops us burning fat, priming us to lay down fat stores for times when food is in short supply. Fasting means our bodies have less work to do, and when insulin isn't circulating, we can start burning the fat stores for energy. Intermittent fasting also improves insulin sensitivity, which is good because we want our bodies to be as sensitive to insulin as possible, so we respond faster and more efficiently. It's one of the key factors in reducing our risk of developing type 2 diabetes.

Many of the health effects discussed here are preventative, so it's harder to see results. But as the 5:2 groups and forums grow, we're getting lots of anecdotal evidence that 5:2 is having a positive effect on a range of conditions, including asthma, menopausal symptoms, arthritis and even snoring.

What about 5:2 and the mind?

Research has shown that fasting may protect against dementia, increase mental sharpness and energy, and even have a positive effect on the chemicals and processes that play a part in depression and other mood disorders.

The evolutionary benefits of fasting on focus and memory are clear: if our ancestors were hungry, it made sense for them to be able to remember where they last found food or to think up a new plan for hunting or trapping prey!

Much of the evidence for the long-term effects on brain chemistry and function is based on animal studies, but these tests can still be useful in determining what the effects may be on humans. In one study, rats and mice genetically engineered to develop dementia, developed the condition sooner when they were fed a diet of junk food, and much, much later than expected when they were put on an intermittent fasting diet.

There's a lot of anecdotal evidence of improvements in mood and focus from people on the 5:2 Facebook group and forums, and this is something I've experienced too. Usually I get really fed up in the winter months, but since starting 5:2 I have more energy than ever and my mood has stayed positive.

Much more research is needed on the effects of fasting on brain chemistry. The role of BDNF (brain-derived neuropathic factor) seems key: low levels of this protein are associated with Alzheimer's, depression and some compulsive behaviours. Fasting may increase levels in the brain, with potentially positive effects. See the Tool Kit section for further reading suggestions (pages 352–353).

How long can I stay on 5:2?

For as long as you like. Many people realise very soon after starting 5:2 that it's a plan we can follow for the rest of our lives, because it feels so easy and natural. Once you reach a healthy weight, you might like to shift from 5:2 to 6:1 (see page 13).

Where can I get more support?

For specific medical issues or questions, be sure to consult your doctor, another specialist or a diabetes nurse.

For general support, the 5:2 forum and the Facebook group

are brilliant – I've never come across such a generous, well-informed bunch. We'd love you to join us!

Find the main forum at the5-2dietbook.com/forums and the Facebook group at facebook.com/groups/the52diet – both are free to join.

A word about words

The words we use affect our thinking – and there's plenty of healthy debate in the 5:2 groups about how we should describe what we're doing. Is 5:2 a diet, a plan, an approach or a way of life? Should we really be calling our Fast Days 'fasts', when we are allowed to eat? And does calling non-fasting days 'Feast Days' encourage us to pig out, or does it simply make us appreciate the food we love?

For this book, I do use the term 'diet' because it's a brief and simply means 'what we eat', but I know it has negative associations for some people. So if 'approach', 'way of eating', 'plan' or 'lifestyle' work better for you, that's fine with me!

Equally, if you'd prefer to think of your Feast Days as Non-Fast Days, Normal Days or (my new favourite) Free Days, that's great. Everything about this diet/approach/way of life is flexible to suit your own needs. It's one of the things that I've found so refreshing after years of restricted meal plans.

What really matters is that you make choices that work for you to help you make changes that, I hope, will be for life!

Enough of the appetiser, it's time for the main course!

2

5:2
FOOD

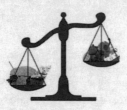

5:2 Fast, Fresh, Delicious

I've always loved cooking. Actually, that's not *quite* true. At school I dreaded Home Economics and produced one of the worst apple jalousie pastry cases my teacher had ever seen. Luckily, I've never felt the need to make an apple jalousie since.

Things improved immensely after I left home, which is lucky for readers of this book, but I do still remember the tricky process of teaching myself to decipher recipes and cook food I actually wanted to eat. So I've worked hard to make these recipes as clear – and as delicious – as possible. All the recipes, including those from our dieters, have been double-tested to make sure they work perfectly every time.

When I started 5:2, I hated the idea of 'diet' food – I'd had my fill of cottage cheese and pineapple on cardboard crisp bread over the years. So at first, I relied on re-heating ready-made soups on Fast Days, but pretty soon I was tempted back into the kitchen to experiment. Of course, I realised that cooking for Fast Days couldn't rely on sploshes of olive oil or dollops of butter.

Instead, I focused on fresh, seasonal produce, clever cooking methods and the most exciting flavours from all around the world. It's been such fun to put together the book I wish I'd had when I started out.

Of course, the recipes aren't just for Fast Days – you'll probably want to make your favourites throughout the week, maybe adding a little extra cheese, oil or meat on a Feast Day.

I really hope the pages of your copy of this book will end up covered in cooking stains and notes or ideas of your own – so feel free to scrawl on the recipes, adapt them, eat breakfasts for dinner or dinners for breakfast. And I'd love to hear what you think – my contact details are at the back of the book!

Before we get cooking, here are a few pointers to help you on your way…

Think Like a 5:2 Cook

Cooking methods

When it comes to 5:2 cooking, there's a compromise to be made between flavour and calories. Steaming and boiling don't involve adding any fats, so they are safe bets calorie-wise. Whereas roasting and frying enhance the flavour of many meats and vegetables, but they do involve using fat (and, therefore, increase the total number of calories).

My compromise is to use a 1-cal cooking spray, which you can buy in most supermarkets, for recipes where frying or roasting is the best option for maximising flavour. These sprays are strange to use at first; you spray them on to a cold pan, and they're white because they're an emulsion of oil and water, with a few other ingredients added in (including alcohol that the makers say evaporates completely during the cooking process). They also help avoid food burning and sticking to the pan.

When I want a little additional flavour, I will use 'real' fats and count the calories – not just in cooking but also in salad dressings (see pages 312–315).

Whether you're using sprays or small quantities of oil or butter, it's usually better to cook at slightly lower temperatures than you're used to, to reduce the risk of burning. This is particularly important for garlic, which can burn very quickly; burnt garlic tastes horrible and will ruin your entire dish. You can also add a little water or lemon juice if food begins to burn or stick.

For roasting, you can use 1-cal cooking spray or a little oil brushed over the surface of your food with a pastry brush (I like the silicone brushes because they're easy to wash). If you wrap food in foil before roasting, you don't always need to add any fat – use herbs or spices to enhance the flavour.

I haven't included 1-cal cooking spray in the calorie counts for the recipes because how much you use depends on the size of the pan and pan temperature. Generally, you'll need two or three sprays (and calories) to mist the surface of a medium-large saucepan and two sprays on each side of the veg, meat or fish that you're planning to roast. An alternative is to get a pump spray and fill it with olive oil, but it will mean you're using more calories and it is harder to monitor.

Fats and oils

One look at the calorie chart on pages 340–349 will confirm how little fat it can take to derail your Fast Day. There are some oils and fats, however, which make up for their calorie count in flavour, even in very small quantities – I'm talking a quarter of a teaspoon. Here is a selection of the oils and fats I use most frequently.

Extra virgin olive oil
I don't use this for cooking because high temperatures reduce its health benefits, but in salad dressings, the flavour makes it worthwhile.

Sesame oil
The strong nutty flavour enhances stir-fries and dressings. I like the toasted sesame oil as it has the most intense flavour.

Coconut oil
This comes in a jar and is actually solid at room temperature, like butter, which means it's easier to control how much you use. It's my new favourite fat – strange as that sounds – because it's very stable at high temperatures and adds a very slight coconut flavour that's really appealing in curries or spicy dishes.

Research also suggests a whole range of health benefits including positive effects on diabetes, brain function and anti-microbial properties. It's even great as a hand cream! You can't say *that* about margarine!

Butter
What? Yes, it's true. I'd never use it on toast on Fast Days – too dangerously tempting – but for cooking, half a teaspoon will add extra flavour and butter is another fat that doesn't deteriorate at high temperatures. Butter has had a bad press, yet in moderation, I think it's one of the good guys. The tricky bit, of course, is the moderation.

In baking, you can use the 'lightest' spreadable butters, which give the buttery taste and moisture but without as many calories as real butter. Check the labels though as calories vary!

On measurements and calorie counting

On your Fast Days, weighing your food is both important and enlightening, especially at first. I have a small digital scale and weigh everything in grams, so I can get very accurate measurements.

You'll be surprised at how much some foods weigh – especially seemingly healthy foods like muesli, where the suggested portion size given on the packaging looks tiny in the bowl. With relatively few calories to play with on Fast Days, it's important to be informed about what each food offers us in energy terms – and energy is what calories measure. Oh, and one small point: what most of us call calories are actually *kilo*calories, which is why nutrition labels use the abbreviation 'kcal'.

Personally, I've found that all that weighing of ingredients affects how I eat on Feast Days, too. I definitely don't weigh food or calorie count (boring!) on non-Fast Days, but the care and attention to what I'm eating rubs off, and the new awareness of portion size is very useful: it's a little re-education in what we need and what we don't.

However careful you are with your measurements, you can never be 100 per cent certain how many calories you're consuming. If you've ever compared the count given for the same ingredient in two calorie counting books or on different websites (or even the same one, in the case of MyFitnessPal), you'll know why. An 'average' onion can be listed as everything from 30–55 calories. Even the measurements per gram can vary, so here are some guidelines.

- Herbs and spices are tricky because we're usually dealing with such tiny quantities. To keep things simple, we haven't counted a few herb leaves used as garnish, a squirt of lemon juice, or a little citrus zest.

- For a handful (10g) of fresh herbs, a tablespoon of chopped herbs (the volume reduces when they're chopped) or a teaspoon or equivalent of dried spices, we've allowed five calories. Chilli peppers also vary in size: allow between two and ten calories for half a small chilli up to a longer fruit.

- Stock for soups can vary. I explain more about these in the 5:2 Extras chapter (see pages 297–323).

- Grated hard cheese, like Parmesan, is difficult to measure in teaspoons as it varies according to how finely it has been grated, so we have always given this in weight.

- In all recipes where there is a range of calorie counts, we've used the lower calorie options to provide the calorie total for the specific dish.

We really have burned the midnight oil comparing and contrasting the measurements of all foods across numerous sources and sites, to try and make the most comprehensive and thorough calorie checker possible. (You can find this at the back of the book on pages 338–348).

I know it seems contradictory to tell you to measure to the last gram in one sentence, and then in the next to mention that calorie counters can be unreliable, but it's best to be upfront!

Of course, manufactured foods are rigorously tested to ensure calorie counts are consistent, but given the choice of ready meals, or home-cooked dishes where I know exactly where and how they are made, I'll take the risk of the odd extra calorie.

Phew . . . time to get cooking.

CHAPTER ONE

Great Starts

ANYTIME BREAKFASTS AND BRUNCHES

My partner always says, 'Breakfast like a king, lunch like a prince, dine like a pauper.' I think, on Fast Days at least, he may be wrong (sorry, R).

Since starting 5:2, I've found that the later in the day I leave eating, the easier I find my Fast Days. It's almost as though eating stimulates my appetite. I asked members of the 5:2 Facebook group the same question. I received 344 replies, and only 65 people said that they always eat breakfast. Many said the same as me: that Fast Days were a doddle since they'd stopped eating breakfast.

But whether you're in my boyfriend's camp or mine, many of the dishes we traditionally see as being breakfast meals are perfect for Fast Days: nutritious, filling and satisfying. I don't mean sugary cereals or even most fruit smoothies because these are very likely to make you hungry again before elevenses. I mean breakfasts and brunches like the ones in this book that contain protein to stave off any hunger pangs.

Many of the recipes feature eggs, a great 'whole' food that will keep you fuller for longer. The concerns about eggs affecting cholesterol in the body have been disproved and for most of us, it's safe to eat as many as we like. Read on for tempting breakfasts you can eat at *any* time of day.

RECIPES

JACQUELINE'S SWAMP JUICE

BANANA OAT MUFFINS

VANILLA GRANOLA POTS WITH BERRY FRUIT COMPOTE

MUSHROOM AND SPINACH OMELETTE MUFFINS

SPEEDY BAKED EGG WITH TOMATO AND HAM

PORTOBELLO MUSHROOM RAREBIT – NAUGHTY AND SKINNY VERSIONS!

HUEVOS 'FASTEROS'

First, one 5:2 dieter shares her tips and recipes in *5:2 Lives*.

5:2 Lives

JACQUELINE'S 'NO DIET' DIET

*The best thing about 5:2 is how easy it is to do.
You just don't feel like you are on a diet.'*

Testing cake and bread recipes is a really tough job, but someone's got to do it. That someone is self-taught food writer Jacqueline Meldrum.

Jacqueline, who lives in Dundee, Scotland, with her husband Graham and three-year old son, Cooper, developed a passion for cooking when she became a vegetarian more than two decades ago. Her inspiring food blog, www. tinnedtomatoes.com, was set up in 2007 and charts her growing love of baking. But all those scrumptious cakes were taking their toll on her waistline.

'In August 2012 I am ashamed to say I weighed a little over 83kg (182 lb). My doctor didn't seem to be concerned about my weight when I had a wellness check-up, but I was. My little boy was two at the time and I still hadn't lost that stubborn pregnancy weight.'

As well as developing recipes for food brands and parenting sites, Jacqueline also hosts the Clandestine Cake Club in Dundee. So a traditional 'diet' was always going to be hard to fit around her work. Then she saw the BBC *Horizon* documentary 'Eat, Fast and Live Longer'.

Jacqueline, who is 42, realised fasting could work for her. 'It was just so inspiring. Here was an easy way to lose weight and to improve health. As an older mum, anything that will keep me healthy and around for my little boy for longer is worth doing.'

Now her blog contains recipes for 5:2 days as well as cakes! She's been losing around 0.45kg (1 lb) a week, but doesn't deprive herself on family celebrations and holidays.

'I took two weeks off at Christmas and New Year and a week off for a holiday, but the good thing is I know I can easily lose any weight I put on after a holiday. I've lost just over 6kg (14 lb) and have gone from a size 16 to a size 14. I feel very energetic and positive.'

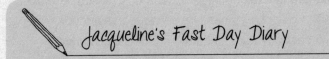

Jacqueline's Fast Day Diary

When I first started 5:2 I spread my calories throughout the day, but I found I was always hungry at night. Now, my typical diet on a Fast Day consists of lots of water during the day, with either soup (70–100 calories), two crisp breads with some Philadelphia Light (80 calories) or a small salad (100 calories) for lunch. I aim to come in under 100 calories at lunchtime, then I drink lots of water until dinner. If I need a wee pick-me-up, I'll have a low-calorie hot chocolate in the afternoon (25 calories).

I always fast on a workday, which I find much easier, as I don't have much time to think about it.

In the evening I'll have a filling meal such as savoury rice with vegetables, a stew or pasta. If I want something simpler, I have two boiled eggs with two slices of toast. If I have calories left over, I typically have an apple or some fat-free Greek yoghurt.

Feast Day Secrets

I don't calorie count on Feast Days, although I do find myself being more aware of the calories in food. I can pretty much eat and drink what I want, without going too crazy.

Favourite Foods

My downfall is definitely cheese and wine. Both are a no-no on Fast Days.

Fast Day Top Tips

- Drink lots of water and keep busy.

- Try to approach the day with a positive attitude and remember that tomorrow you can eat what you like.

- If you need a sweet treat, jelly beans are only four calories each.

The Best Thing About 5:2

The best thing about 5:2 is how easy it is to do. You just don't feel like you are on a diet. There's none of the predictable thinking about food constantly (well not too much, but I am a food blogger, after all) and being miserable.

JACQUELINE'S SWAMP JUICE

Jacqueline says: 'This is a really lush, nutritious smoothie that I invented when I went back on to the 5:2 Diet at the start of 2013. I whizzed it up in my wonderful new blender. Unfortunately, the plastic plug wasn't in the lid and I had decorated the cupboard doors a lovely green before I realised. Luckily, I didn't lose too much smoothie! It also got the thumbs up from my son, Cooper. I added some milk and yoghurt to the leftover smoothie and he enjoyed that too.'

Makes 4 small glasses
Calories per glass: 98
Preparation time: 5 minutes

30g baby spinach leaves *8 cals*
handful fresh mint leaves *5 cals*
1 ripe avocado (around 150g) *235–285 cals*
400ml fresh apple juice (not from concentrate) *144–196 cals*

1. Rinse the spinach and mint leaves and pat dry with a clean tea towel.

2. Remove the peel and stone from the avocado and cut the flesh into rough pieces.

3. Whizz all the ingredients in a blender until smooth. You may like to add a few ice cubes if your blender is strong enough and you prefer your smoothie ice cold. Add a splash of water if you prefer your smoothie to have a thinner consistency.

4. Serve and enjoy, feeling smug and healthy!

Kate says: I love all the recipes on Jacqueline's blog, but the colour of this smoothie and the fun name really jumped out at me! I'm always worried that smoothies will give me a sugar rush on Fast Days, which will mean I am hungry again within an hour, but this one doesn't do that thanks to the mix of fruit and vegetables.

BANANA OAT MUFFINS

Muffins on a Fast Day? But these, my friends, are no ordinary muffins. Pop one in your bag with a flask of coffee for a breakfast on the go that will help you resist the sugary temptations of your local barista. The seeds and oats help keep you full, and they're as low in sugar as we can make them without losing the taste. Add whatever seeds you have to hand. They freeze well: cool completely and freeze in a plastic box for up to one month. Defrost fully before serving.

Makes 12
Calories per muffin: 219
Preparation time: 15 minutes
Cooking time: 20–25 minutes

100g rolled oats *355 cals*
50g wholewheat flour *155 cals*
150g plain white flour *503 cals*
2 tsp baking powder *10 cals*
1 tsp bicarbonate of soda *5 cals*
¼ tsp salt
75g muscovado sugar *300 cals*
4 large very ripe bananas, mashed *480 cals*
1 large egg, beaten *100 cals*
4 tbsp light olive oil *540 cals*
2 tbsp pumpkin or sunflower seeds or a mix *175–184 cals*

1. Preheat the oven to 180°C/350°F/Gas mark 4. Line a 12-hole muffin tin with paper cases.

2. Mix together the oats (keeping a tablespoon aside for the topping), flours, baking powder, bicarbonate of soda, salt and sugar.

3. Mix together the mashed bananas, egg and oil and then pour into the dry oat and flour mix and fold together.

4. Spoon into the prepared muffin cases and scatter the top of each muffin with the reserved oats and the seeds. Bake for 20–25 minutes, until brown and slightly springy to touch.

VANILLA GRANOLA POTS WITH BERRY FRUIT COMPOTE

Granola is one of my favourite things – baking the ingredients gives it a crunch that makes it a cut above common-or-garden muesli. The addition of a roasted fruit and berry compote is irresistible and works well if you want your breakfast/brunch to be one of the main events on Fast Days – and, of course, it's yummy on Feast Days too. Why not bake a batch on a Sunday to see you all the way through the week? The compote will keep in the fridge for up to three days.

Vanilla Granola
Makes 350g (7 x 50g servings)
Calories per 50g serving: 231
Preparation time: 10 minutes
Cooking time: 35 minutes

1 tbsp vegetable oil *135 cals*

5 tbsp maple syrup (or agave syrup) *191 cals*

1 tsp vanilla extract *12 cals*

150g jumbo rolled oats *533 cals*

3 tbsp mixed seeds, such as sunflower, sesame and pumpkin *270 cals*

45g whole blanched almonds, roughly chopped *275 cals*

75g mix of dried cherries, sultanas and chopped dried apricots *203 cals*

Berry Fruit Compote

Makes 3 servings
Calories per serving: 76
Preparation time: 5 minutes
Cooking time: 18 minutes

2 ripe peaches or nectarines *102 cals*
1 tbsp agave syrup or honey *44–60 cals*
finely grated zest ½ orange and a squeeze of juice *5 cals*
1 cinnamon stick
75g blackberries *30 cals*
35g blueberries *20 cals*
75g raspberries *29 cals*

1. Preheat the oven to 150°C/300°F/Gas mark 2. To make the granola, mix together the oil, maple syrup and vanilla in a bowl. Add the rest of the ingredients except the dried fruit and stir together.

2. Spread over a baking sheet lined with non-stick baking paper and bake for 20 minutes. Add the fruit, mix well and bake for a further 10–15 minutes, until golden brown. Leave to cool completely before storing in an airtight jar for up to a month.

3. For the compote, turn up the oven to 180°C/350°F/Gas mark 4. Remove the stones from the peaches or nectarines, cut into wedges and place on a large baking tray. Drizzle over the agave syrup, orange zest and juice, and add the cinnamon stick. Bake for 15 minutes or until the fruit is tender.

4. Add the berries and bake for a further 2–3 minutes to soften slightly. Tip the hot fruit into a bowl and leave to cool.

5. To serve, layer the granola with the fruit compote in a glass or small bowl — you can add a dollop of fat-free natural yoghurt, too, if you desire (but remember to count the calories for this). You could also take a pot of this to work with you.

MUSHROOM AND SPINACH OMELETTE MUFFINS

These are the perfect breakfast (or lunch, or supper) on the go. They're easy to cook *and* to reheat, and they look really cute, too. A little Parmesan goes a long way . . . You can use different fillings like ham, tomato or chopped peppers to vary the flavours.

Makes 6
Calories per muffin: 83
Preparation time: 10 minutes
Cooking time: 20 minutes

   1-cal cooking spray
   125g chestnut mushrooms, sliced *16 cals*
   1 clove garlic, chopped *4 cals*
   100g spinach, chopped *25 cals*
   4 large eggs, beaten *400 cals*
   30ml skimmed milk *11 cals*
   10g Parmesan cheese, finely grated *42 cals*
   salt and pepper

1. Preheat the oven to 200°C/400°F/Gas mark 6. Spray a non-stick frying pan with 1-cal cooking spray, add the mushrooms, season well and fry over a high heat for 3–4 minutes, until they start to turn golden.

2. Add the garlic and fry for a further minute and then add the spinach and leave to wilt for 1 minute. Remove from the heat and set aside to cool. Drain off any excess liquid.

3. Whisk together the eggs, milk and half the Parmesan in a bowl. Season well and then stir in the mushroom and spinach mixture.

4. Line a 6-hole muffin tin with paper cases or simply lightly grease each hole with 1-cal cooking spray. Divide the egg mixture between the cases and sprinkle the tops of the muffins with the rest of the Parmesan.

5. Bake for 15 minutes, or until puffed up and golden. Serve while still hot. (If the muffins aren't all going to be eaten straight away, allow them to cool and then keep them in a plastic box in the fridge for 3–4 days. Reheat the muffins in the microwave for 25 seconds.) If you don't have a microwave, reheat in the oven at 180°C/350°F/Gas mark 4 for 5 minutes or until warmed through.

SPEEDY BAKED EGG WITH TOMATO AND HAM

Call me eccentric, but I have a particular passion for food served in ramekins. Maybe because I know that everything inside that little pot is *mine, all mine*. This is a surprisingly low-cal breakfast for one with lots of savoury goodness. And for those days when you're in a tearing hurry, you can also microwave it in moments.

Serves 1
Calories per serving: 138
Preparation time: 5 minutes
Cooking time: 12–15 minutes

    1-cal cooking spray
    ½ tomato, chopped *8cals*
    1 slice lean smoked ham, chopped *5 cals*
    1 egg *78 cals*
    1 tbsp half-fat crème fraîche *26 cals*
    5g Parmesan cheese, finely grated *21 cals*
    salt and pepper

1. Preheat the oven to 180°C/350°F/Gas mark 4. Lightly grease a ramekin with 1-cal cooking spray.

2. Place the tomato and ham in the base of the ramekin. Carefully crack in the egg, spoon over the crème fraîche, season well and scatter with the Parmesan.

3. Bake for 12–15 minutes, until the white has set but the yolk is still runny. Serve immediately.

Microwave method

1. Prepare as above, but make sure you carefully pierce the egg yolk with the prong of a fork or a toothpick (otherwise it will explode). Cover with a lid or some kitchen paper and cook on high for 30 seconds.

2. Check the eggs and then cook for a further 20 seconds. The white should be set and the yolk still runny. If not, cook for another 10 seconds. Don't be tempted to microwave in a one-minute burst, as it will cook too quickly. An overcooked egg is the fastest way to ruin your Fast Day!

PORTOBELLO MUSHROOM RAREBIT –
Naughty and Skinny Versions!

I can't believe I've got this far without mentioning how much I love cheese. Finding a cheese fix on my Fast Days was a top priority for me, and so I've adapted this classic recipe by substituting high-cal bread for saintly but tasty portobello mushrooms – the kind that are as big as a hamburger. Of course, if you have the calories to spare, you could also make this with a small slice of wholemeal bread. Or the mix will keep in the fridge for a day, so you could have the second portion on your Feast Day, served on toast with a fried egg on top. I've added a second, 'skinny' version for an even lower-cal cheese hit. Shirley Conran said, 'Life's too short to stuff a mushroom.' This is the proof that she was wrong!

Naughty Rarebit
Serves 2 as a main, or 4 as a small snack
Calories per serving: 228 (as a main)
Preparation time: 5 minutes
Cooking time: 6–8 minutes

> 4 x 80g portobello mushrooms, wiped clean *83 cals*
>
> 1-cal cooking spray
>
> 1 egg *78 cals*
>
> 75g mature Lancashire cheese, finely crumbled or grated *279 cals*
>
> 2 tbsp stout or semi-skimmed milk *6–12 cals or 7 cals*
>
> 1 tsp English mustard *9 cals*

splash Worcestershire sauce (or the veggie equivalent, made
    without anchovies)
salt and pepper

1. Preheat the grill to medium. Place the mushrooms on a baking tray
   lined with foil and spray with 2 or 3 sprays of 1-cal cooking spray. Grill
   stalk side facing up for 4–5 minutes, or until the mushrooms have just
   softened (the biggest mushrooms may take a little longer).

2. Meanwhile, prepare the rarebit mix. Beat the egg with a fork in a small
   bowl. Add the cheese followed by the rest of the ingredients and mix
   well. Season with salt and pepper.

3. Spoon the egg mixture on top of the mushrooms (if they've released a
   lot of liquid, pour this off the baking tray first). Place back under the grill
   for 2–3 minutes, until the cheese mixture puffs up and browns, but make
   sure it doesn't burn.

4. Drain off any further cooking liquid from the mushrooms before serving
   alongside something with a strong flavour, like a peppery rocket or
   watercress salad.

Variations: Instead of using portobello mushrooms, you could
use 320g smaller mushrooms (42 cals) sliced and spread in a
layer. Try the same mixture in two halves of a small pepper
(30 cals). Add a chopped spring onion (1–2 cals) and a couple
of cherry tomatoes (6–10 cals) to the pepper halves and cook
as instructed above.

Skinny Rarebit

Serves 1
Calories per serving: 96
Preparation time: 5 minutes
Cooking time: 7 minutes

2 x 80g portobello mushrooms, wiped clean *42 cals*
1 teaspoon of English mustard *9 cals*
2 level tbsp Philadelphia Light (any flavour) *45–48 cals*
salt and pepper

1. Grill the mushrooms as above, then spread the tops with the mustard, using the back of a teaspoon. Divide the cheese between the mushrooms in an even layer. Grill for 2 minutes. Season and serve while still hot.

Variations: As this version is so low in cals, you could serve with a 25g slice of wholemeal toast (55 cals) or a Warburton's Thin (100 cals for both slices).

You could use pesto instead of mustard (1 teaspoon of bottled pesto is around 23 calories, depending on brand), and top with a 25g pre-sliced piece of light Cheddar (60 extra cals), crumbled over the mushrooms.

HUEVOS 'FASTEROS'

The Spanish introduced chickens to Mexico in the sixteenth century and soon Huevos Rancheros (ranch-style eggs) became a national dish. This brunch (or anytime) dish is super-satisfying. I've taken some liberties with the authentic version to make allowances for a Fast Day but there are extra options you can add, calories allowing. You can easily multiply this recipe to serve more people – you'll just need a larger frying pan.

Serves 1
Calories per serving: 230
Preparation time (not including sauce): 2 minutes
Cooking time: 7 minutes

¼ portion Mexican Tomato Sauce (see page 307) *30 cals*
1 egg *78 cals*
1 small corn tortilla *117 cals*
handful coriander leaves (or any fresh green herbs, e.g.
    oregano or chives) *5 cals*
salt and pepper

1. Preheat the oven to 140°C/275°F/Gas mark 1. Reheat the Mexican sauce in a small frying pan with a lid. When it's warmed through, make a small well in the middle and break the egg into it.

2. Put the lid on top of the pan and cook over a medium heat for about 3½–4 minutes, until the egg white is cooked and the yolk is still runny. Meanwhile, warm the tortilla on a plate in the oven for 2–3 minutes.

3. When the egg is cooked, use a spatula to carefully place it on top of the tortilla, spooning the Mexican sauce along with it. Season with salt and pepper. Add any of the optional toppings, below, then scatter over the coriander leaves to serve.

Optional toppings:

½ baby avocado, flesh cut into chunks *approx. 80–90 cals*

50g refried beans heated in microwave or small pan *45–50 cals*

15g low-fat feta cheese, crumbled (not authentic but oh so good!) *27 cals*

5:2 Know-How:

THE STORE CUPBOARD

Fresh produce is great, but keeping the store cupboard well
stocked means you'll always have something on hand for those
days when you haven't time to shop – or when you make
a tactical decision to stay out of the supermarket and avoid
temptation. If you've ever been a Guide or a Scout, you know it
makes sense to 'Be Prepared'. Check out the herbs and spices
list in the Fast Day Flavours Know-How section (see pages
127–131 for more ideas).

THE WORKTOP

1-cal cooking spray, olive oil, sesame oil, coconut oil
See the oils section under Think Like a 5:2 Cook (page 37).

Sea salt and black pepper
Keep these handy at all times. I have a pepper grinder and a
pinch-pot of coarse sea salt. Avoid using too much salt, but if
you're cutting down on processed foods – which are the main
source of salt in our diets – you can afford to use a little to
enhance flavours.

Vinegars
See the Fast Day Flavours Know-How section (pages 127–131).

THE CUPBOARD

Baked beans
Half a tin on toast is an easy, low-cal Fast Day lunch or supper.

Basmati rice
Rice isn't an ideal choice for Fast Days, but basmati rice has the least dramatic effect on blood sugar so if you do want rice (rather than the very tasty Cauliflower Rice, see pages 303–304), brown basmati is the one to choose.

Couscous
Faster than rice, and easy to control portion size.

Crispbreads/oatcakes
Ryvita or similar crispbreads can give you a lower-calorie crunch than bread, and oatcakes are useful for the same reason.

Cup-a-soups/miso soup
Good for a lower-calorie snack when you need something more substantial than herbal tea.

Dried mushrooms
These add loads of flavour in soups or veggie dishes for very little effort!

Low-sugar jellies
The saviour of many a sweet-toothed 5:2 newbie. They're sweet and very low in calories to satisfy a craving. You can

either buy the individual pots or, more cheaply, make up your own. Be aware that gelatin is not suitable for vegetarians.

Low-sugar squash/diet drinks
Helpful if you get bored with water on Fast Days. See page 289 for a note about sweeteners.

Nuts and seeds
Nuts and seeds are high in nutrients but also high in calories. A small quantity will give crunch and flavour, but measure carefully.

Olives
A flavourful snack and ingredient. Read the label to check calories and avoid those preserved in oil or stuffed with cheese for Fast Days.

Sun-dried tomatoes (dried)
An intense hit of sunshine and the Med. The dried ones are lower in calories than those that are preserved in oil. If the oiled ones are all you can find, drain them *very* well before use.

Tinned soups
These are often lower-calorie than 'fresh' soups and a great comfort food.

Tinned sweetcorn
Great uncooked in salads or as a speedy side vegetable. Sweetcorn is, however, relatively high in calories for a vegetable so measure carefully.

Tinned tomatoes

The most fuss-free base for a great soup or sauce. I buy ready-chopped plum tomatoes for speed.

Tomato purée

Excellent for adding flavour to all kinds of stews and soups.

Tortillas/flatbreads

Plastic wrapped tortillas have a longer shelf life than bread and are good for packed lunches.

Zero or shirataki noodles

See page 323 for more information.

THE FRIDGE

Cheese:
  Light halloumi
  Ricotta
  Light Greek-style salad cheese/feta
  Philadelphia Light

I tend to avoid most low-fat foods, but these are the most acceptable ones as far as I'm concerned. Low-fat halloumi still fries well, the ricotta is naturally lower in fat than other cheeses, and feta-style cheeses are so flavourful (and salty) that you'll barely notice the reduction.

I am also a fully signed-up Philly-fan, as I do find their Light version creamier than other brands. However, I draw the line at the Extra-Light variety, as I don't like the texture. You may disagree!

Eggs
If you like them, they are filling and nutritious. Buy medium or even small eggs rather than large, you won't notice the difference.

Lemons (or lemon juice)
Indispensable for adding flavour or sliced with hot water as a refreshing drink. I do use ready-squeezed lemon juice when I'm in a hurry.

Low-fat crème fraîche/quark/yoghurt
Pick your favourite to add richness as a topping for soups or hot dishes, and to serve with fruit desserts.

Pre-prepared foods
This book is all about making your own meals, but keeping an emergency fresh soup or lower-calorie ready meal in the fridge will do no harm for those days when you don't have the energy to cook. I won't tell if you won't . . .

Quorn
A very low-fat veggie food made from a form of fungus. The sausages or burgers are usually lower-calorie than the bread-crumbed dishes.

Spring onions

Faster than a normal onion if you snip them into a pan or salad with kitchen scissors.

Wafer-thin ham or turkey

Great for sandwiches and salads.

THE FREEZER

Bananas

I freeze unpeeled over-ripe bananas, either wrapped in foil or placed in a freezer bag, to use in smoothies (or cakes). They turn very mushy when thawed.

Berries

Raspberries and blueberries freeze beautifully. Stir them into yoghurt or use them in smoothies. You can also buy frozen berry mixes.

Home-made lollies

Make ice pops and lollies in a mould using low-cal squash for guilt-free sweetness in the summer. Add a few berries for texture!

Leaf or chopped spinach

For when you don't want to prepare fresh leaf spinach.

Peas, sweetcorn

Frozen just after picking, these hang on to their vitamins and are quick and easy to prepare.

Prepared butternut squash

I have had too many near-death experiences with cutting butternut squash to risk it when I am in a hurry; these are my back-up plan.

Roasted Mediterranean veg/grilled peppers

These surprised me. They reheat well and are tasty for when you haven't had chance to grill your own peppers.

White fish fillets (e.g. cod, haddock, pollock, coley)

For a really fast and low-calorie supper.

CHAPTER TWO

Super Soups

TO KEEP YOU FULL ON FAST DAYS

Soup has saved many a 5:2 Faster from giving in on a wintry day. And it's a great, light choice in summer, too. I've included lots of soup recipes in this book because they are so filling and adaptable, like a great big hug in a bowl.

Scientists have also shown that soup keeps you satisfied for longer, compared to eating the same calories in a solid meal. Adding liquid means the stomach stays full for a longer period – and that stops the stomach cells sending a message to your brain to tell you it's time to eat again. A *very* good thing on a Fast Day.

Add that to the fact that soup is perfect for work packed lunches – and that being a whizz with soup will impress your friends and family (somehow producing home-made soup leads to compliments that far exceed the effort involved) and you will agree that soup is absolutely, well, *super*.

RECIPES

KIRSTY'S BUTTERNUT SQUASH AND SWEET POTATO SOUP

RUBY SOUP

BRANDIED MUSHROOM SOUP
(with chestnuts when you feel like it)

HEARTY TUSCAN BEAN SOUP

SPRING VEGETABLE AND PESTO MINESTRONE

SPICY CHICKEN, COURGETTE, BASIL AND ORZO SOUP

PANCH PHORAN TOMATO AND RED LENTIL SOUP

UDON NOODLE MISO SOUP

BEEF PHO

GAZPACHO

5:2 Lives

KIRSTY'S FASTING CURE

'I have been telling anyone who will listen that this is life changing.'

Ceramic artist Kirsty Badham was diagnosed with an underactive thyroid in August 2012. The symptoms were really affecting her life. They included painful joints, low energy, dry skin and depression.

'I felt particularly low around Christmas, and I had been struggling to get my medication right. I was overweight because I have always loved food and have never found it easy to stop when I feel full.'

Kirsty, who is 43 and lives in Bedfordshire, began following 5:2 in the first week of 2013. Almost immediately she noticed a tremendous difference.

'Since I began 5:2, all the symptoms have subsided without any change to my medication levels. I have much more energy, my mood has lifted considerably and the pain in my joints has all but disappeared.'

That, combined with weight loss of 6kg (13 lbs) in the first eight weeks, has turned Kirsty into a 5:2 fan. And, like many following the plan, she's also noticed a significant difference in her attitude to eating. 'Doing this has made me connect with the feeling of being hungry and accept it as a positive thing.

I now enjoy the feeling of being satisfied and stopping when I'm full.'

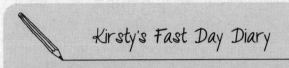

Kirsty's Fast Day Diary

If I have two meals, I have a homemade soup (120 calories) at 2 p.m. and a salad with some form of protein like grilled chicken or prawns (around 250 calories) in the evening. Extra calories are used up on things like Bovril drinks and perhaps some hummus with veggies to fill the gaps! I have started to avoid carbs and milk on Fast Days and have done a couple of fasts just eating in the evening.

Feast Day Secrets
I have slowed down how I eat and reduced portion sizes. I also think much more carefully about how I 'spend' my calories and value the food I eat, rather than eating low-value/high-calorie foods absentmindedly.

Favourite Foods
It has to be a good old roast chicken dinner!

Fast Day Top Tip
* Try not to weigh yourself too much and instead go on how good you feel. It's not all about losing weight. Look at it as a complete lifestyle change rather than just a diet.

The Best Thing About 5:2

I can't stop smiling ☺ and I have been telling anyone who will listen that this is life changing – probably boring them silly with the science of it! Maybe I need to redo the sales pitch, but if nothing else it certainly gets their attention when I tell them I've lost 6kg (13 lb) in eight weeks!

KIRSTY'S BUTTERNUT SQUASH AND SWEET POTATO SOUP

Kirsty says: 'This soup is quick and so simple. Just throw it all in a pan, whizz it up in a blender and you're done! It is a gorgeous orange colour. The velvety texture and appealing colour brightens up your most trying Fast Day and it's really filling.'

Serves 4
Calories per serving: 182
Preparation time: 15 minutes
Cooking time: 25 minutes

  1-cal cooking spray
  1 onion, peeled and cut into small chunks *38 cals*
  200g peeled butternut squash, cut into small chunks *80 cals*
  200g peeled sweet potato, cut into small chunks *180 cals*
  2 medium carrots, peeled and cut into small chunks *68 cals*
  1 tsp curry powder *5 cals*
  100g no-soak red lentils, rinsed *330 cals*
  1 litre vegetable stock (or 1 litre water with 2 tsp Marigold
      bouillon powder) *25 cals*
  salt and pepper

1. Spray a large non-stick saucepan with 1-cal cooking spray (or you can use half a teaspoon of coconut oil, which will add 21 calories but goes well with the spices).

2. Add the onion and allow to soften over a medium heat for 2 minutes. Stir in the butternut squash, sweet potato, carrots and curry powder, and cook for 5 minutes.

3. Add the lentils and stock and bring to the boil. Cover with a lid and simmer for about 20–25 minutes, until the vegetables are soft.

4. Remove from the heat and blend the vegetables in the pan with a stick blender, adding 50–100ml of water if necessary to loosen the consistency. If you don't have a stick blender, use a jug blender. Season, to taste with salt and pepper and serve. You can also freeze this soup in individual portions.

Kate says: This is such a comforting recipe with lots of potential for varying the flavours. Next time, I'm going to try Thai curry paste instead of curry powder, and a splash of coconut milk for an Eastern-inspired version.

RUBY SOUP

I ♥ beetroot, and it ♥ me right back with all its cardiovascular goodies. Yes, beetroot gets the blood flowing. Research shows that the nitrates it contains can lower blood pressure, increase blood flow to the brain and muscles and enhance athletic performance. Plus, it contains vitamin C, fibre, potassium, folate (iron) and antioxidants. Cooking beetroot does reduce its nitrate content but however you eat it, this is a super-powered veg. The colour of this soup alone makes it a Fast Day treat! I've given two great serving options – spicy horseradish or tangy feta-style cheese. Both contrast beautifully with the soup's earthy flavour.

Serves 4
Calories per serving (without topping): 82
Preparation time: 10 minutes (less with food processor)
Cooking time: 15 minutes

    250g fresh or vacuum-packed beetroot (not in vinegar!) *108 cals*
    1 medium dessert apple *80 cals*
    1-cal cooking spray
    1 red onion, peeled and chopped *38 cals*
    1 clove garlic, chopped or crushed *4 cals*
    1 tsp whole cumin *5 cals*
    400g tin chopped tomatoes *72 cals*
    1 tbsp cider vinegar or balsamic vinegar *2–20 cals*
    700–750ml vegetable stock (or 750ml water with 2 tsp
        Marigold bouillon powder) *20–24 cals*

2 fresh bay leaves
2 sprigs thyme or lemon thyme, plus extra to serve
salt and pepper

1. Grate or dice the beetroot and apple. (A food processor comes in very handy for this, and will reduce some of the pink staining to your hands!)

2. Spray a small non-stick saucepan with 1-cal cooking spray, then cook the onion over a medium heat for 2 minutes. Reduce the heat to low and add the garlic and cumin and cook for a further 2 minutes. If it starts to stick to the bottom of the pan, add a dash of water or squirt of lemon juice.

3. Add the beetroot and apple and mix together so the vegetables are combined. Then add the tomatoes, vinegar, stock, bay leaves and thyme.

4. Bring the mixture to a simmer, cover the pan with a lid and cook for 8–10 minutes until the beetroot and apple are cooked.

5. Remove from the heat and remove the bay leaves and thyme sprigs. Use a stick blender or jug blender to blend the vegetables to a smooth consistency. Season to taste with salt and pepper.

6. Serve with either of the two suggested toppings below, or simply scatter over some fresh herbs – chopped parsley or snipped chives go very well with this soup. (Extra portions can be frozen or kept in the fridge before the toppings are added.)

Suggested Toppings

1. Mix 1 level tablespoon of low-fat fromage frais (*25 cals*) per serving into a bowl with grated, fresh or bottled, horseradish to taste (around half a teaspoon per serving/*9 cals*). Spoon into the centre of the soup and stir.

2. Crumble 10g low-fat feta cheese (*18 cals*) per serving over the top of the warm soup – my favourite.

Variation: Try this recipe with shredded red cabbage (75g is 20 calories) instead of the apple. Use balsamic vinegar instead of cider vinegar.

BRANDIED MUSHROOM SOUP
(with chestnuts when you feel like it)

Mushroom soup can be either a delight or a dull, sludgy mess. I experimented with maxing out the luxury for minimum calories with two fancy French additions: chestnuts and cognac. The chestnuts and brandy make me feel festive, but this soup is not just for Christmas. The quantity of brandy is tiny, and you could use sherry instead, or leave it out completely. You can omit the chestnuts too. I've tasted the soup with and without the brandy and chestnuts side by side. Both are excellent, the former is just rather richer. I prefer the full-on version; my other half prefers the more frugal soup. It's your choice.

Serves 2
Calories per serving: 143 with the brandy and chestnuts;
   48 without
Preparation time: 10 minutes
Cooking time: 15–20 minutes

  1-cal cooking spray
  1 onion, peeled and chopped *38 cals*
  1 clove garlic, crushed or finely chopped *4 cals*
  200g mixed mushrooms, sliced (I like a mix of chestnut and
      shiitake for robust flavour) *26 cals*
  1 tbsp brandy or dry sherry (optional) *31 cals or 22 cals*
  grated nutmeg
  100g chestnuts, either vacuum-packed chestnuts or unsweetened
      chestnut purée (optional) *160 cals*

6g dried mushrooms, e.g. porcini or mixed mushrooms soaked
    in 150ml boiling water *15 cals*
550–600ml chicken or vegetable stock (or 600ml water with
    1 tsp Marigold bouillon powder) *12–20 cals*
3 sprigs fresh thyme
salt and pepper

To serve

1 tbsp low-fat crème fraîche per serving *25 cals*
fresh thyme or other fresh herbs (chives work well), chopped

1. Spray a medium non-stick saucepan with 1-cal cooking spray. Heat the
   pan over a medium heat and fry the onion for 2 minutes. Turn the heat
   down a little, add the garlic and cook for a further 2 minutes.

2. Add the mushrooms and fry for about 3–4 minutes. Add the brandy and
   a little grated nutmeg. Stir in the whole chestnuts, if using, and cook for
   another minute.

3. If the dried mushrooms are gritty, strain them through a sieve, keeping
   the soaking liquid for flavour. Pick out the mushrooms, and chop or tear
   them into smaller pieces. Add these to the pan, along with the soaking
   liquid, the chestnut purée, if using, the stock and the thyme sprigs.

4. Increase the heat and bring to the boil, then reduce to a simmer, cover
   and cook for 10 minutes.

5. Remove from the heat and remove the thyme stalks. Use a stick blender
   or jug blender to blend to a smooth consistency. If you like some texture,
   remove some of the mushrooms with a slotted spoon before blending,
   then add back to the mix and stir through. You may need a little more

liquid for the chestnut version, so add a splash of water until you get the consistency you like.

6. Season, to taste, and serve with a dollop of crème fraîche and a scattering of herbs.

Ideas: If you use the vacuum-packed chestnuts, slice any leftover chestnuts and use them in stir-fries or added to recipes like the Mushroom Stroganoff or Beef and Ale Stew (see pages 246–247 or 142–143). They're good as a snack, too (25g are 40 cals).

HEARTY TUSCAN BEAN SOUP

Italian food doesn't have to revolve around pasta or pizza, and this hearty soup is a great example of filling rustic food. The addition of Parmesan cheese and a clever trick with some crumbly Parma ham gives it a fab savoury kick, but you could simply sprinkle fresh herbs on top to cut the calories.

Serves 4
Calories per serving: 136 with Parmesan and Parma ham;
    110 without
Preparation time: 15 minutes
Cooking time: 20 minutes

  1-cal cooking spray
  2 slices Parma ham (optional) *62 cals*
  1 onion, peeled and finely diced *38 cals*
  2 medium carrots, peeled and finely diced *68 cals*
  2 sticks celery, finely diced *12 cals*
  400g tin mixed beans, drained *230 cals*
  2 large ripe tomatoes, chopped *40 cals*
  1.2 litres hot fresh chicken or vegetable stock (or made from
      good-quality stock cubes) *30 cals*
  75g savoy cabbage, core removed, shredded *20 cals*
  10g Parmesan cheese, freshly grated (optional) *42 cals*

1. Preheat the grill to medium. Lightly oil a baking sheet with 1-cal cooking spray. Place the Parma ham on the baking sheet and grill for about 3–4 minutes, until crisp. Remove and set aside to cool.

2. Spray a large non-stick saucepan with 1-cal cooking spray, add the onion, carrots and celery and a splash of water to help the vegetables steam and fry over a medium heat for 3 minutes.

3. Stir in the beans, tomatoes and hot stock, bring to the boil, cover with a lid and simmer for 5 minutes. Stir in the cabbage and simmer for 2 minutes, or until just tender.

4. Spoon into serving bowls and scatter with the Parmesan and crumble over the crispy Parma ham, if using.

SPRING VEGETABLE AND PESTO MINESTRONE

Every Italian family will have a different recipe for minestrone, but adding pesto is typical of the northern region of Liguria. This filling soup sings with flavour and is one of my favourites – with its green veg and touch of red from the tomatoes, this is definitely springtime in a bowl. It's best made with fresh pesto.

Serves 4
Calories per serving: 127 with cheese; 106 without
Preparation time: 20 minutes
Cooking time: 15 minutes

1-cal cooking spray
1 small onion, peeled and finely chopped *38 cals*
2 sticks celery, finely chopped *12 cals*
1 carrot, peeled and finely chopped *34 cals*
100g baby leeks, finely sliced *22 cals*
1 courgette (170g), finely chopped *34 cals*
2 cloves garlic, finely chopped *8 cals*
2 tsp sundried tomato paste *20 cals*
1.2 litres hot fresh chicken or vegetable stock (or 1.2 litres water
    with 3 tsp Marigold bouillon powder/good-quality chicken
    stock cube e.g. Kallo) *30–36 cals*
2 ripe tomatoes, skinned and chopped *32 cals*
75g green cabbage or cavolo nero, finely shredded *20 cals*
40g thin vermicelli noodles, broken into pieces *132 cals*
2 tsp fresh basil pesto *42 cals*
20g Parmesan cheese, finely grated (optional) *84 cals*
salt and pepper

1. Spray a large non-stick saucepan with 1-cal cooking spray, add the onion, celery, carrot, leeks, courgette and a splash of water. Gently fry over a low heat for 3–4 minutes, or until softened but not coloured. Add the garlic and sundried tomato paste and fry for a further minute.

2. Add the hot stock and tomatoes and bring to the boil. Add the cabbage and noodles, season well and simmer for 2–3 minutes, until the cabbage and noodles are just tender.

3. To serve, divide the soup between bowls, drizzle with a little pesto and scatter with the grated Parmesan, if using.

SPICY CHICKEN, COURGETTE, BASIL AND ORZO SOUP

Chicken soup deserves its nourishing reputation. When it's combined with vegetables, basil and orzo (a tiny pasta that looks like rice) then you have a bowl of nutritious deliciousness. This soup freezes very well; freeze it without fresh herbs.

Serves 4
Calories per serving: 134
Preparation time: 20 minutes
Cooking time: 1 hour

  1-cal cooking spray
  1 carrot, peeled and finely chopped *34 cals*
  2 sticks celery, finely chopped *12 cals*
  1 leek (180g), finely chopped *40 cals*
  1 onion, peeled and finely chopped *38 cals*
  2 chicken thighs, skin removed *212 cals*
  2 bay leaves
  50g orzo *165 cals*
  1 small courgette, finely chopped *25 cals*
  2 tbsp chopped fresh basil or parsley *10 cals*

1. Spray a large non-stick saucepan with 1-cal cooking spray. Add the carrot, celery, leek and onion and fry over a medium heat for 3–4 minutes, or until softened. Add a splash of water to help the veggies steam.

2. Add the chicken thighs, bay leaves, and enough water to just cover everything (about 1.2 litres). Bring to the boil and then simmer gently for 45 minutes, until the chicken is cooked through.

3. Remove the chicken from the pan, shred the meat and set aside. Discard the bones.

4. Add the orzo to the pan and cook for 3 minutes. Add the shredded chicken and courgette and simmer for 3 minutes, or until the courgette is tender. Scatter with the chopped herbs before serving.

PANCH PHORAN TOMATO AND RED LENTIL SOUP

My favourite all-rounder soup. I adapted this from the Tomato and Lentil Soup in *The 5:2 Diet Book*, using a panch phoran spice blend I'd bought. The recipe is incredibly versatile and low maintenance. Just prep the veg, add the lentils and do something else for 20 minutes, then come back and tuck in!

Serves 2
Calories per serving: 118
Preparation time: 3 minutes
Cooking time: 25 minutes

    1-cal cooking spray
    1 onion, peeled and chopped *38 cals*
    pinch chilli flakes
    1 tsp panch phoran spice blend *5 cals*
    450–500ml vegetable or chicken stock (or 500ml water with
        1 tsp Marigold bouillon powder) *12 cals*
    2 tbsp dried red lentils *99 cals*
    400g tin chopped tomatoes *72 cals*
    large handful fresh coriander leaves, to taste *10 cals*
    salt and pepper

1. Spray a medium non-stick saucepan with 1-cal cooking spray. Fry the onion, chilli and spice mix over a medium heat for 2–3 minutes, adding a dash of water if necessary, to prevent the onion mix from sticking.

2. Add the stock, lentils and tomatoes to the pan and bring to the boil. Use less stock for a thicker, heartier soup. (You could start with 450ml stock

and then add a little water at the end to achieve the consistency you like.) Cover and simmer for 20 minutes, or until the lentils are soft.

3. Stir in the coriander, cook for a minute and then remove from the heat and blend with stick blender until smooth. If you don't have a stick blender, use a jug blender. Season to taste, with salt and pepper and serve.

Variations: Experiment with your favourite spices: whole coriander or cumin seeds are lovely, or add some ground ginger and turmeric. This freezes very well so why not double up the portions for your next Fast Day – the ultimate in Fast Food!

UDON NOODLE MISO SOUP

I think of miso as the Japanese version of Marmite, not that they taste anything like the same, but they're both intense pots of serious flavour. Miso is made from fermented soybeans or rice, and miso soup is traditionally served for breakfast. I particularly recommend the brown rice version, which keeps for a year in the fridge (add hot water for instant soup, or really great with salmon as a marinade). This noodle soup is deeply flavoured and packed with healthy ingredients, including vegetables and tofu. Tasty *and* virtuous.

Serves 1
Calories per serving: 226
Preparation time: 10 minutes
Cooking time: 10 minutes

300ml boiling water
1 tbsp miso paste *17 cals*
2cm piece fresh root ginger, peeled and grated *2 cals*
35g tenderstem broccoli florets *11 cals*
1 baby pak choi, leaves separated *13 cals*
50g enoki mushrooms or exotic mushrooms *13 cals*
50g silken tofu, drained and cut into small cubes *43 cals*
½ tsp soy sauce *2 cals*
75g udon or soba noodles *103 cals*
½ tsp sesame oil *22 cals*

1. Pour the boiling water into a medium saucepan and mix in the miso paste. Add the ginger and broccoli and simmer for about 3–4 minutes, or until tender.

2. Add the pak choi, mushrooms, tofu and soy sauce and warm through for 1–2 minutes.

3. Cook the noodles according to the packet instructions and then drain and tip into a serving bowl.

4. Pour the soup and vegetables over the noodles and drizzle with a little sesame oil.

BEEF PHO

This *really* doesn't look, smell or taste like diet food; it's a meal in a bowl, thanks to the noodles, and it'll fill your kitchen with lovely aromas. If you want something just as fragrant but a little lighter, you can always leave out the noodles. The beef is sliced just 2–3mm thick, so it cooks the moment it hits the hot stock and is beautifully tender in the finished soup. There are no calories included for the aromatics – the lemon grass, ginger and lime leaves – as they are removed before serving. This soup is so good you'll probably want to double up the quantity – the spiced stock will keep for up to 4 days in the fridge.

Serves 1
Calories per serving: 260 with noodles; 183 without the
   noodles
Preparation time: 5 minutes
Cooking time: 15 minutes

   300ml fresh beef stock *15–30 cals*
   1 stick lemon grass, bashed and chopped
   3cm piece fresh root ginger, peeled and sliced
   1 red chilli, sliced
   2 Kaffir lime leaves
   35g thin egg noodles (optional) *77 cals*
   75g mixed sugar snap peas and baby sweetcorn, sweetcorn
      halved lengthways *25 cals*
   75g lean beef fillet, very thinly sliced (see above) *132 cals*
   small handful bean sprouts *10 cals*

salt and pepper
fresh coriander leaves, to garnish

1. Pour the stock into a medium saucepan, add the lemon grass, ginger, half the chilli (reserve the rest to garnish) and the lime leaves. Bring to the boil, then simmer, covered, for 10 minutes. Strain through a sieve into a clean saucepan and discard the aromatics.

2. Add the noodles, if using, and cook for 2 minutes. Add the sugar snap peas and baby sweetcorn and cook for a further 2 minutes. Season the beef, add to the soup and heat through for 1 minute.

3. Pour into a bowl, gently stir through the beans sprouts and scatter with the remaining sliced chilli and the coriander.

Variation: Try this with 75g cooked and shredded chicken (124 cals) instead of the beef or, for a veggie version, use 75g tofu (65–139 cals), a few dried or fresh shitake mushrooms (8 cals) and vegetable stock (10 cals).

GAZPACHO

I couldn't see the appeal of chilled soup till we moved to Spain and I tasted *real* Gazpacho for the first time. Now this refreshing, low-calorie dish brings back memories of sunset suppers accompanied by a cold, dry sherry. This recipe uses sherry vinegar so you get the flavour, without the booze. I'm a chilled soup convert and if you try this, you will be too. You could leave out the croûtons to reduce the calories to the minimum, but this soup is so saintly and healthy that surely you deserve a little crunch? Take a look at the photo to see how appetising it looks!

Serves 4
Calories per serving: 110 with croutons and garnish;
  81 without
Preparation time: 10 minutes

600g deep red, ripe tomatoes, chopped *120 cals*
1 large clove garlic, chopped *4 cals*
1 red pepper, seeded and chopped *30 cals*
½ cucumber, peeled and chopped *10 cals*
1 tsp caster sugar or sweetener (you may not need this if the
    tomatoes are very ripe and sweet) *15–0 cals*
2 tbsp sherry vinegar *10–15 cals*
1 tbsp olive oil *135 cals*
salt and pepper

For the garnish (optional)

> 1 slice granary bread, cut into 0.5cm cubes *59 cals*
>
> 1 tsp olive oil *45 cals*
>
> Red, yellow, orange and green peppers, cucumber and spring
> onions, all finely chopped (as a guide, use 2 strips of each
> colour pepper cut into 0.5cm cubes, 4cm piece of cucumber
> cut into 0.5cm cubes, and 4cm piece spring onion – per
> person) *12–15 cals*

1. Place the tomatoes, garlic, red pepper and cucumber in a blender and blend until smooth. Season well, add the rest of the ingredients and blend again. Pass through a sieve into a large jug and chill for at least an hour.

2. For the croûtons, fry the cubes of bread in the oil over a medium heat until golden.

3. Pour the chilled soup into bowls and garnish with the croûtons, chopped peppers, cucumbers and spring onions, if using.

5:2 Know-How:

TOOLS OF THE TRADE

I have a passion for kitchen gadgets. A serious passion.
When the Lakeland kitchenware catalogue arrives, I am in
seventh heaven as I try to resist buying a lemon pod, a dish
squeegee or some Stack-a-Boxes (actually, the boxes are the
best things I've ever bought from the brochure). My eyes are
definitely too big for my kitchen cupboards, though, and I am
trying to streamline. So here is a list of my Tools of the Trade
for 5:2 cooking: the Must-Haves, the Nice-to-Haves and the
Up-to-Yous. I reckon all larger appliances need to pass the
worktop test: will you use it often enough (at least once a
week) to justify a place on your worktop? If not, you might
like to give it a miss.

MUST-HAVES

Blender (stick or jug)
I've had the same little Moulinex Turbomix for years. It takes up
hardly any space and is a whizz when it comes to blending
soups in the pan. Look for one with a decent motor and a
robust-looking design. You can get them from under £10 to
over £100 with all sorts of attachments – ask yourself honestly
how often you'd use the extras. A jug blender makes smoother

soup but means more washing up – buy one with a jug that can go in the dishwasher!

Box grater

Cookware shops sell dozens of variations of graters but a box grater is the most versatile and will handily keep all your gratings confined.

Digital scale

A must for measuring down to the last gram or fraction of an ounce. You can use it with any bowl, adding ingredients as you go, and can pick one up for less than £5.

Measuring spoons

Quicker than the scales and ideal for dressings. Buy basic; I still use the grey plastic ones I bought when I kitted out my first flat.

Non-stick pans

Non-stick surfaces make cooking with little or no fat so much easier. One medium saucepan and a frying pan should be enough for most situations and I'd advise buying the best you can afford, as they'll last longer and the coating is less likely to flake off. To go with them, you need wooden or silicone spatulas that won't scratch the pan's surface.

Plastic boxes/freezer bags

For cooking in bulk and freezing extra portions of soups, main dishes and baked items. As I mentioned, Lakeland Stack-a-

Boxes take up less space in cupboards and avoid scrambling around trying to find the right lid to fit the right box. Freezer bags are good for soup or sauces, though use two for strong-smelling food to stop other items being tainted. No one wants a fishy ice-cube in their G&T.

Vegetable peeler

I prefer a Y-shape design to a conventional potato peeler. The Good Grips ones feel very comfortable to use. They are good for peeling veg, making courgette 'pasta' (see pages 321–322), and for *very* thin shavings of cheese or chocolate.

Very sharp knife

No need for a knife-block full of different sizes. A medium cook's knife that fits well in your hand will serve you well.

NICE-TO-HAVES

Food processor

Great if you're going to use it. Not so great if it's going to end up in the cupboard. I bought a small one (a Magimix Mini Plus), which has an even smaller bowl for very small quantities of garlic or nuts. It stays on the worktop and that reminds me to use it all the time to grate, slice and chop.

Mandolin

Not the musical instrument, but a nifty tool that's brilliant for shaving off super-thin slices of veg or fruit. It also makes you feel very cheffy. I had to watch a few YouTube videos before I got the knack. Choose one with a hand-guard, as those razors are, well, razor-sharp.

Soup-maker/all-in-one cooker and blender

I almost bought the Rolls Royce of processors, the Vitamix, which costs about the same as a holiday and will cook soup and perform about a hundred different other functions. Then I calmed down and realised it would take up most of my worktop and how hard was it to make soup in a pan anyway? However, many people in the 5:2 Facebook group swear by them for making fruit juices, soups and many other dishes.

UP-TO-YOUS

Actifry

A machine that can fry anything – including great chips – with minimal oil. To be honest, deep-frying doesn't feature in many Fast Day meals so this isn't an essential, but many forum members do like the results!

Breadmaker

Again, bread isn't a great choice on a Fast Day so not an essential for 5:2. Plus the smell of fresh bread can be too tempting . . .

Potato ricer

One forum member swears by hers for making lower fat toppings for pies, not just from normal potato but also butternut squashes, sweet potatoes and other root vegtables. It creates a very smooth mash. It will also purée fruit – mash doesn't feature much in my life but if you love it, this is a cheap buy.

Slow cooker

Great for tender meat dishes and vegetable stews and economical to run. Does it pass the worktop test?

Zester and melon baller

I don't use either of these *that* much but the zester saves my knuckles and the melon baller creates dinky spheres of all kinds of produce for salads. The baller is also great for getting flesh out of veg you want to stuff, like courgettes. Not essentials but these tools are inexpensive and don't take up too much room in the kitchen drawer.

CHAPTER THREE

Hot Stuff

TO SPICE UP FAST DAYS

I love curry. My aunt and uncle introduced me to the joys of a chicken korma at their local Indian restaurant in Merseyside when I was little. I loved the décor, the poppadoms, the sauces and the orange sorbet in its shell.

Poppadoms are not on the menu here, but spices definitely are. Adapting dishes to make up for the lack of buttery ghee or rich but fatty coconut milk means balancing the spices so you get all the depth of flavour but without the calories.

RECIPES

LIZZIE'S HARIRA

THAI GREEN, RED, YELLOW
(or whatever colour you like) **CURRY**

JERK CHICKEN WITH COCONUT RICE AND
PINEAPPLE CHILLI SALSA

KATE'S SAAG PANEER

RAITA

LAMB KOFTA IN PITTA POCKETS WITH FETA,
CUCUMBER SALAD AND MINTY YOGHURT SAUCE

ASIAN SEARED BEEF WITH RAINBOW STIR-FRY

VEGETABLE BIRYANI

STICKY INDONESIAN PORK STIR-FRY

SKINNY CHILLI CON CARNE

5:2 Lives

MEET MR AND MRS 5:2

Want that treat today? Think of all the good things you can have tomorrow.'

A husband and wife dieting together might sound like a recipe for disaster. But for food-lovers Kevin and Lizzie Baker from Wiltshire, 5:2 is an unqualified success. Between them, they lost 45kg (100 lb) in less than six months.

When they started in September 2012, Lizzie had a BMI of 28.5. Kevin's was 43.7, which put him in the obese category. As an account manager for a drinks market research company, the beer testing, overseas travel and conference banquets were taking their toll. And Lizzie's home cooking wasn't helping either.

Lizzie says: 'Since we moved to the country, we'd begun eating far too many farm-shop treats but weren't doing as much walking as we wanted.' They adopted Guinness, a rescue border collie, but found keeping up with a lively dog was hard work. 'Kevin actually caused some damage and was told to rest his legs to heal them, but that wasn't going to help essential weight loss. Something had to be done.'

At 55 and 51, Lizzie and Kevin were very aware of the health issues surrounding excess weight. Their fathers both died of strokes and their mothers had circulatory problems. When

Lizzie's doctor suggested she started taking statins to manage her cholesterol, she decided to try 5:2 instead. The Bakers fast every Monday and Friday with impressive results. Kevin has lost 35kg (77 lb) and his BMI is a massive 10 BMI points lower, while Lizzie now has a lower BMI of 25 and healthy cholesterol levels.

Their clothes fit them better too, although Kevin's trousers now look like a teenager's, so big he can wear them in a 'low-slung, saggy-baggy style!' They're both able to walk the dog for hours without any pain, and their daughter is now on 5:2 with her partner, for the health benefits. Plus, Lizzie says they're both more rested. 'Kevin's snoring, which had reached walrus proportions, has nigh on disappeared, so he must be sleeping better because of it.'

Kevin and Lizzie's Fast Day Diaries

Kevin has breakfast at 8 a.m., which usually consists of a bowl of cereal and milk with a probiotic yoghurt drink. He skips lunch. Lizzie doesn't eat until late lunch – anytime between 2 p.m. and 4 p.m. – when she'll have a large portion of salad with a little ham or fish. Lizzie always drinks a couple of cups of coffee with skimmed milk (she needs those!) and as she feels the cold on winter Fast Days she tops up with one or two hot mugs of marmite.

Kevin and Lizzie eat dinner together between 6 p.m. and 7 p.m. when they'll have a large portion of homemade soup.

They make a 'bucketful' on Monday and keep the rest until Friday. They've not yet repeated a variety of soup!

Feast Day Secrets

We don't count calories at all on Feast Days but we have found our appetites have adjusted as we go along. Kevin's 'quick treat' grabbed at the railway station might have consisted of a caramel macchiato, a panini and a cheesecake; now he'll probably just have the caramel macchiato.

We never use or buy any low-calorie or diet food options. The closest we get to low-cal is semi-skimmed milk. The Sunday roast is always cooked in homemade dripping. Our house has an Aga and to justify the expense of it, almost everything is made from scratch including bread. We have over 30 jars of homemade jams and preserves in the cupboard – and Lizzie makes a mean clotted cream fudge! The other day we made our own peanut butter – now that was a revelation. Without 5:2 there'd be no hope for us!

Favourite Foods

Kevin: Pasta, curry, macaroni cheese, pizza, spotted dick (compulsory on my birthday!).

Lizzie: CHOCOLATE! Also, coffee, all sorts of cheeses (you really can't beat a tingly Cheddar on a digestive biscuit) and nuts (cashews, pistachios, pecans and macadamias).

Fast Day Top Tips

Kevin: It is a challenge at first but it gets easier; it will work! Want that treat today? Think of all the good things you can have tomorrow.

Lizzie: Try a bit of distraction therapy. I might spend the day looking at recipe books planning something really good to eat for the next day.

The Best Thing About 5:2

It's NOT a diet in the restrictive sense, so you can do it forever and it's not like you're wearing a hair shirt. You don't have to deny yourself at all in the long run.

LIZZIE'S HARIRA

Lizzie says: 'Harira seems a particularly apt dish for Fast Days because it is the traditional soup eaten after sunset during Ramadan. I'm not a Muslim but just thought this sounded rather special, and it certainly tasted it when I made it. This version is a mix of the best bits of different recipes given to me by former colleagues. It can be completely vegetarian too.'

Serves 4–6
Calories per serving: 284–189
Preparation time: 15 minutes
Cooking time: 30–35 minutes

   100g dried red lentils, rinsed *330 cals*
   120g tinned chickpeas, drained and rinsed *130 cals*
   1 stick celery, sliced *6 cals*
   1 carrot, peeled and diced *34 cals*
   400g tin tomatoes *72 cals*
   ¼ tsp chilli powder or a fresh one, deseeded and chopped
      3 cals
   1 tsp turmeric *5 cals*
   1 tsp ground ginger or 1 tbsp grated fresh root ginger *5 cals*
   1 tsp ground cinnamon *5 cals*
   pinch cayenne pepper
   handful chopped fresh coriander leaves, to serve *5 cals*
   salt and pepper

For the soup base

300g skinless chicken breasts or thighs, with fat trimmed off, cut into bite-sized pieces *495 cals*

1 onion, peeled and chopped *38 cals*

2 cloves garlic, chopped *8 cals*

1–1.2 litre vegetable or chicken stock or water *0–35 cals*

bunch fresh thyme sprigs

good pinch salt

1. Put all the ingredients for the soup base in a large saucepan. Bring to the boil over a high heat, then reduce the heat and simmer for about 10–15 minutes.

2. Add all the other ingredients (apart from the chopped coriander) and bring back to the boil, before covering and simmering for a further 20 minutes, until the lentils and chicken are cooked through.

3. Remove the thyme sprigs, season to taste with salt and pepper and serve sprinkled with the coriander.

Kate says: This dish is so hearty and warming and you don't miss the chicken in the veggie version because the spices work so well together. Definitely a soup to relish on wintry evenings – but I'll be making it into the summer months too.

THAI GREEN, RED, YELLOW (or whatever colour you like) CURRY

I love Thai curries but traditional recipes are too high in fat – and calories – for a Fast Day. Reduced-fat coconut milk helps, but it is not as rich, so you need to use more spices to compensate. You can buy frozen Thai herbs, or jars containing blends of lemon grass, garlic, chilli and basil if you don't have time to chop and grate. And don't stress too much if you're missing an ingredient.

This is a veggie version made with tofu, but the variations at the end of the recipe for chicken and prawns also work brilliantly. Experiment with your favourite veg and aim for a mix of colours and textures. I cook and chop at the same time, adding the densest vegetable first (broccoli or cauliflower) and tipping more veg into the pan when it's ready. Keep any leftover curry covered in the fridge overnight to eat the next day.

Serves 3 generously
Calories per serving: 170
Preparation time: 10 minutes, plus marinating
Cooking time: 18 minutes

  200g firm tofu, drained and cut into small cubes *170–370 cals*
  1 tsp light soy sauce (or fish sauce for non-veggies) *3 cals*
  1 lime *20 cals*
  2 tsp grated fresh root ginger *5 cals*
  2 Kaffir lime leaves
  ½ stick lemon grass, bashed

2 tsp Thai curry paste (choose from green, red or massaman; check the label for fish sauce if you're vegetarian) *about 16 cals*

1 red chilli, ½ finely chopped, ½ sliced into rounds *4–8 cals*

1-cal cooking spray

5 spring onions, sliced *6 cals*

2 cloves garlic, crushed *8 cals*

125g broccoli, broken into florets *40 cals*

1 yellow or red pepper, seeded and sliced *30 cals*

1 courgette, sliced on the diagonal *34 cals*

75g shitake mushrooms, any larger ones sliced in half *19 cals*

200ml reduced-fat coconut milk (check the label) *about 150 cals*

small handful fresh basil or coriander leaves, torn or roughly chopped *5 cals*

1. First marinate the tofu. In a shallow bowl, mix together the soy or fish sauce, the juice from half the lime (save the other half for serving), the ginger, lime leaves, lemon grass, curry paste and the finely chopped chilli. Add the tofu pieces and toss lightly to coat in the marinade. Leave in the fridge for an hour, or overnight, for the flavours to develop.

2. Heat a few sprays of 1-cal cooking spray in a large non-stick saucepan (or you can use half a teaspoon of coconut oil, which will add 21 calories but goes well with the spices). Fry the spring onions over a medium-high heat for 2 minutes, then reduce the heat, add the garlic and fry for a further minute. Add the tofu and marinade to the pan and fry for 2 minutes.

3. Add the veg. Fry for 1–2 minutes to coat the veg in the marinade.

4. Pour in the coconut milk and mix gently. Simmer for 10–12 minutes, until the vegetables are tender (you may prefer to cook them for a little

longer, depending on how crunchy you like your veg). Remove the lime leaves and lemon grass.

5. Serve the curry with the remaining lime half cut into wedges. Sprinkle with the remaining chilli slices and garnish with a little basil or coriander. This is excellent with a portion of Cauliflower Rice (see pages 303–304).

Variation: Replace the tofu with the same weight of raw king prawns (*130 cals*) or small chunks of chicken breast (*330 cals*). Prepare and cook as above, but fry the chicken for 4–5 minutes before adding the vegetables, and make sure it's cooked through before serving.

JERK CHICKEN WITH COCONUT RICE AND PINEAPPLE CHILLI SALSA

Cooking with jerk seasoning always makes me think of hot bank holiday weekends at the Notting Hill Carnival, with the smell of barbecued meats and the sound of reggae in the air. Caribbean food doesn't get anything like the attention of other cuisines but the allspice and scotch bonnet peppers in jerk seasoning give meat – or even tofu – a seriously hot hit. The rice and salsa work beautifully to make this a generous main meal for two, but for a lighter dish for a Fast Day you could serve the chicken with steamed greens.

Serves 2
Calories per serving: 481 with rice; 316 without
Preparation time: 15 minutes, plus marinating
Cooking time: 25 minutes

> 2 tbsp jerk paste (such as Bart's) *60 cals*
> 2 x 100g skinless chicken breasts, fat trimmed *330 cals*
> 1-cal cooking spray
> 150ml reduced-fat coconut milk *110 cals*
> 150ml boiling water
> 100g wholegrain rice, rinsed (optional) *330 cals*
> 75g tinned kidney beans, rinsed and drained *70 cals*
> salt and pepper

For the salsa (optional)

100g fresh pineapple, finely chopped *50 cals*
½ red chilli, deseeded and finely chopped *2–4 cals*
2 tbsp chopped fresh coriander *10 cals*

1. Spread the jerk paste over both sides of the chicken breasts. Place on a baking sheet lightly oiled with 1-cal cooking spray and leave to marinate for 10 minutes.

2. Heat the grill to medium and grill the chicken for 5 minutes on each side, or until cooked through.

3. Pour the coconut milk and boiling water into a small pan. Add the rice, bring to a simmer, cover with a lid and cook for 20 minutes. Top up with more water as necessary.

4. Add the kidney beans, season well and cook for 5 minutes, or until the rice is tender.

5. For the salsa, mix the pineapple with the chilli and coriander.

6. Serve thick slices of the chicken with the coconut rice and pineapple salsa on the side.

KATE'S SAAG PANEER

This is my kryptonite when I go out for a curry. The smoothness of the spinach, combined with the chewy cubes of spiced cheese, mean no meat is required. I wanted to make a lower-calorie version, which would still feel like a treat on Fast Days – and I've cracked it! With a packet of paneer in the fridge and some frozen spinach in the freezer, you will always have this on standby. Double the quantities if you want to take it to work: it'll keep, covered, in the fridge for two days (add the crème fraîche when you reheat it). This version is fairly mild, so up the chilli and ginger for more of a kick.

Serves 1 as a main or 2 as a side dish
Calories per serving: 246 with crème fraîche, 220 without
Preparation time: 10 minutes
Cooking time: 10 minutes

    50g paneer, cut into 1cm cubes *about 150 cals, (check label)*
    1-cal cooking spray (or ½ tsp coconut oil, *21 cals*)
    ½ onion, peeled and finely chopped *19 cals*
    1 clove garlic, finely chopped *4 cals*
    2cm piece fresh root ginger, grated *2 cals*
    ½ small red or green chilli, deseeded and finely chopped
        2–4 cals
    125g frozen spinach *31 cals*
    lemon juice, to taste, about 10ml *2–4 cals*
    salt and pepper
    1 tbsp half-fat crème fraîche (optional) *26 cals*

For the spice mix *10 cals*

½ tsp chilli flakes or powder
½ tsp turmeric
½ tsp ground cumin
½ tsp salt
½ tsp garam masala

1. Mix together the ingredients for the spice mix in a small bowl. Place the paneer cubes in the spice mix and coat well.

2. Heat a small non-stick saucepan over a medium heat with either 1-cal cooking spray or *half* the coconut oil. Add the cheese and spices and cook for 5 minutes, moving the cheese around the pan to stop it burning. (I like mine just this side of burned, so it is browned on the outside.)

3. Pop the cooked paneer back in the bowl, then either re-spray the pan with 1-cal cooking spray or add the rest of the coconut oil. Fry the onion, garlic, ginger and chilli over a low heat for 3 minutes, making sure they don't burn.

4. Add the spinach and cook over a medium heat for 2–3 minutes, or until the spinach is cooked. Add a little water to stop it sticking to the pan.

5. Put the paneer back in the pan, along with some lemon juice (1–2 teaspoons) and heat for a minute. Season with salt and pepper.

6. If serving immediately, remove from the heat and stir in the crème fraîche, if using. Serve with raita (see page 116) and Cauliflower Rice (see pages 303–304).

Variation: To make Matter Paneer (with peas and tomatoes), add 2 large chopped tomatoes (*32 cals*) instead of the spinach and fry for 2 minutes, before adding 80g frozen peas *(54–60 cals)* and 100ml water. Cook for 5 minutes and then add lemon juice, to taste. You won't need the crème fraîche. Total calories when made with 1-cal cooking spray: 275 cals.

RAITA

The perfect side dish for any spicy curry is a yoghurt-based raita. You can use this as the basic recipe and add whatever other ingredients you like: grated carrot works well, as does cucumber, though add this shortly before you serve it, otherwise it can make the mix watery.

Serves 4
Calories per serving: 35
Preparation time: 5 minutes

> ½ red onion, peeled and diced *19 cals*
> handful fresh coriander leaves, chopped *5 cals*
> handful fresh mint leaves, chopped *5 cals*
> 200ml natural or fat-free Greek yoghurt *110–130 cals*
> salt and pepper

1. Mix all the ingredients together in a serving bowl. Season with salt and pepper and stir well before using. It will keep, covered, in the fridge for a couple of days, although the herbs may lose their freshness.

LAMB KOFTA IN PITTA POCKETS WITH FETA, CUCUMBER SALAD AND MINTY YOGHURT SAUCE

Forget kebabs, koftas are where it's at. This is a really filling dish with great depth of flavour – perfect for serving to friends who don't know you're on a diet! Freeze the uncooked koftas for up to a month and defrost fully before cooking, as below. They'll also keep cooked in the fridge for a couple of days.

Serves 4
Calories per serving: 443; 280 without pitta or feta
Preparation time: 30 minutes, plus chilling
Cooking time: 10 minutes

400g lean minced lamb *832 cals*
½ red onion, peeled and finely chopped *19 cals*
3cm piece fresh root ginger, peeled and grated *3 cals*
2 cloves garlic 8 cals
1 tsp ground cumin *5 cals*
1 tsp ground coriander *5 cals*
1 red chilli, deseeded and finely chopped *4–8 cals*
1 egg, beaten *78 cals*
2 tbsp finely chopped fresh mint *10 cals*
1-cal cooking spray
40g low-fat feta cheese, cubed (optional) *72 cals*
salt and pepper
4 wholemeal pitta breads or flatbreads, warmed, to serve
   (optional)*145 cals per pitta*
2 Little Gem lettuces, shredded, to serve *25–30 cals*

For the minty yoghurt sauce

200ml fat-free natural yoghurt *110–130 cals*
small bunch fresh mint, finely chopped *10 cals*
½ tsp cumin seeds, toasted
½ cucumber, peeled and deseeded *10 cals*

1. For the koftas, mix together the lamb, onion, ginger, garlic, spices, egg and mint in a bowl and season well. Shape into walnut-sized balls and place in the fridge to chill for 20 minutes.

2. Heat the grill to high. Place the lamb balls on a baking sheet, spray with a little 1-cal cooking spray and grill for 8–10 minutes, or until golden brown and cooked through.

3. For the minty yoghurt sauce, mix the yoghurt with the mint and cumin seeds. Grate 6cm cucumber, squeeze out the excess water, and add to the yoghurt and season well. Cut the remaining cucumber into small cubes and set aside. Season the cucumber and the feta.

4. To serve, split open a warmed pitta bread, scatter with shredded lettuce, spread with a little minty yoghurt, top with the hot lamb balls and then scatter with chopped cucumber and feta.

ASIAN SEARED BEEF WITH RAINBOW STIR-FRY

Somewhere over the rainbow . . . there's a dream of a dish that's surprisingly low in calories. The sirloin steak rightly takes centre-stage in this stir-fry that is bound to get a standing ovation on Fast Days. It serves four, enough for Dorothy, the lion, the tin man and the scarecrow. Or, alternatively, for you and some friends.

Serves 4
Calories per serving: 183
Preparation time: 20 minutes
Cooking time: 15 minutes

1 large clove garlic, crushed *4 cals*
juice of ½ lime, plus extra wedges to serve *10 cals*
1½ tbsp light soy sauce *4 cals*
1 tsp light brown sugar *15 cals*
3cm piece fresh root ginger, peeled and grated *3 cals*
1 long red chilli, thinly sliced *4–8 cals*
200g sirloin steak *300–350 cals*
2 tsp sesame oil *90 cals*
2 carrots, peeled and cut into ribbons with a vegetable peeler *68 cals*
1 red onion, peeled and sliced *38 cals*
150g Tenderstem broccoli, trimmed *48 cals*
100g mix sugar snap peas and baby sweetcorn *34 cals*
75g frozen edamame beans *98 cals*
100g pak choi, leaves separated *17 cals*
salt and pepper

1. First make a dressing by mixing together the garlic, lime juice, soy sauce, sugar and ginger and chopped chilli in a bowl, then set aside.

2. Heat a griddle or frying pan over a high heat. Brush the beef all over with half the sesame oil and season with salt and pepper. Griddle for 2 minutes on each side, then remove and leave to rest for 5 minutes covered with foil. Slice into thin strips and keep covered.

3. Meanwhile, heat the remaining sesame oil in a wok over a high heat. Add the carrot, onion and broccoli and stir-fry for 2 minutes. Add the sugar snap peas, baby sweetcorn and the edamame beans and pak choi leaves. Add a splash of water (to help steam the veg) and stir-fry for a further 3 minutes.

4. Divide between 4 bowls, top with the beef and drizzle over the dressing. Serve with extra lime wedges.

VEGETABLE BIRYANI

There's something very festive about biryani. I love the colour of the spiced rice contrasting with the vegetables and the lovely herb and nut topping. Rice is quite calorie-dense but here the fragrant grains are the main event. If you like fruit, you can also add a tablespoon of sultanas to the rice before baking (this will add 42 calories).

This dish makes a great family meal. Serve it with Raita (see page 116) for everyone and poppadoms and naan bread for the rest of the family. You *can* make smaller portions though it's a little fiddly using smaller quantities of vegetables. It's best eaten immediately after cooking as it won't taste as nice reheated.

Serves 4
Calories per serving: 253
Preparation time: 15 minutes
Cooking time: 35 minutes

    130g cauliflower, cut into small florets *33 cals*
    2 carrots, peeled and cut into small cubes *68 cals*
    75g fine green beans, trimmed and halved *20 cals*
    1-cal cooking spray
    1 large onion, peeled and thinly sliced *38 cals*
    2 tbsp hot Madras curry paste *16–30 cals*
    200g brown basmati rice *660 cals*
    2 tsp black or white mustard seeds *30 cals*
    700ml hot vegetable stock *20–25 cals*
    50g frozen peas *35 cals*

juice of 1 lemon *19 cals*

2 tbsp chopped fresh coriander or flat-leaf parsley leaves
10 cals

10g toasted flaked almonds *63 cals*

1. Preheat the oven to 190°C/375°F/Gas mark 5. Steam the cauliflower, carrots and beans for 4 minutes, or until just tender but with a bit of bite. Set aside.

2. Spray a pan with a little 1-cal cooking spray, add the onion and fry over a medium heat for 5 minutes, or until softened and turning golden brown.

3. Add the curry paste and fry for a further minute. Add the rice and mustard seeds and mix well to coat.

4. Tip into a lightly oiled ceramic baking dish, pour over the hot stock and stir together. Cover tightly with foil and bake for 20 minutes or until the rice is tender and the liquid is almost absorbed. Stir in the steamed vegetables and cook for 5 minutes more.

5. Stir in the frozen peas and lemon juice and season, to taste. Scatter over the coriander and flaked almonds and serve.

STICKY INDONESIAN PORK STIR-FRY

The delicious sticky marinade takes its sweetness from the ketjap manis, a thick and syrupy spiced soy sauce used in Indonesian cooking. This is one of the few dishes in the book that can't really be frozen or adjusted down, portion-wise, but if you do all the preparation in one go, and refrigerate half overnight, you will have two meals for two in double quick time!

Serves 4
Calories per serving: 204, 247 including rice
Preparation time: 20 minutes, plus marinating
Cooking time: 10 minutes

  2 tbsp ketjap manis *60 cals*
  1 tbsp light soy sauce *3 cals*
  juice of ½ lime, plus extra to serve *10 cals*
  1 clove garlic, finely chopped *4 cals*
  3cm piece fresh root ginger, peeled and grated *3 cals*
  400g pork tenderloin, cut into 3cm cubes *560 cals*
  1-cal cooking spray
  1 red chilli, sliced *4–8 cals*
  4 spring onions, finely sliced *4–8 cals*
  1 red and 1 yellow pepper, seeded and cut into wedges
    60 cals
  225g tin bamboo shoots, drained *16 cals*
  8 baby pak choi, leaves separated *80 cals*
  2 tbsp chopped fresh coriander leaves *10 cals*
  50g steamed jasmine rice, to serve (optional) *174 cals*

1. Mix the ketjap manis, soy sauce, lime juice, garlic and ginger in a bowl. Add the pork, stir to coat and leave to marinate for up to 30 minutes.

2. Spray a wok or large non-stick frying pan with 1-cal cooking spray and heat over a high heat. Cook the pork for about 3 minutes, or until browned all over.

3. Add the chilli, spring onions, red and yellow peppers and any leftover marinade, and fry for 2–3 minutes, or until the pork is cooked through.

4. Add the bamboo shoots and pak choi and heat through for 1–2 minutes. Stir through the coriander and serve with steamed jasmine rice, if desired.

Variation: You can replace the pork with cubed tofu for an equally fragrant vegetarian version with a lower calorie count.

SKINNY CHILLI CON CARNE

It's no wonder this Mexican dish is so popular, so far from home. It's perfect for wintry evenings – and this skinny version means you really don't have to miss out on Fast Days. Serve with Cauliflower Rice for you (see pages 303–304) and normal rice for them! You can also freeze individual portions for up to three months so this is a great dish for batch cooking.

Serves 4
Calories per serving: 246
Preparation time: 15 minutes
Cooking time: 55 minutes

1-cal cooking spray
1 onion, peeled and finely chopped *38 cals*
2 sticks celery, finely chopped *12 cals*
1 carrot, peeled and finely chopped *34 cals*
2 cloves garlic, finely chopped *8 cals*
2 green chillies, deseeded and finely chopped *8–16 cals*
400g extra-lean minced beef *480 cals*
1 tsp ground cumin *5 cals*
2 tsp sweet paprika *10 cals*
2 fresh tomatoes, chopped *32 cals*
400g tin chopped tomatoes *72 cals*
1 tbsp tomato purée *4 cals*
200ml boiling water
1 cinnamon stick
1 fresh bay leaf

300g tinned kidney beans, drained and rinsed *280 cals*
salt and pepper

For the garnish (optional)
chopped fresh coriander leaves and low-fat soured cream or
half-fat crème fraîche (a tablespoon of the soured cream will
add 15 calories and crème fraîche is 26)

1. Spray a non-stick saucepan with a little 1-cal cooking spray. Add the onion, celery and carrot and season well. Add a splash of water to help the vegetables steam and cook over a low heat for 3–4 minutes. Stir in the garlic and chillies and cook for another minute.

2. Add the beef, mix together gently and fry for 5–6 minutes, or until golden brown. Add the spices and fry for a further minute.

3. Stir in the fresh and tinned tomatoes and leave to cook down for about 5 minutes. Stir in the tomato purée.

4. Pour over the boiling water and add the cinnamon stick and bay leaf. Bring to the boil, reduce the heat and simmer for 30 minutes, stirring occasionally, until the sauce is beginning to thicken.

5. Add the kidney beans and cook for 5–10 minutes to allow the beans to soak up the flavours.

6. Remove the cinnamon stick and bay leaf (yes, this is correct to remove before serving) and serve scattered with chopped coriander and a dollop of soured cream or crème fraîche, if using, on the side.

5:2 Know How

FAST DAY FLAVOURS

The best thing I ever did, to add flavour to my cooking, was to buy a masala dabba. It's an airtight circular tin with a transparent lid and seven little pots inside. You fill the pots with the seven spices you use most often, and use the tiny spoon to add to your cooking as you go. So you have none of that struggling to open different jars with greasy hands, or spilling herbs everywhere as you try to measure out a teaspoon.

My tin contains turmeric, ground ginger, cumin seeds, coriander seeds, cardamom pods and chilli flakes. In the central pot I keep cloves, a cinnamon stick and bay leaves. All ready for action – it improved my cooking overnight! You can buy your own masala dabba online for around £10.

The list below shows even more ways to enhance Fast Day Flavours and keep those taste buds entertained.

Capers
These funny little nuggets of flavour, preserved in jars, work well with fish or roasted vegetables. You either love them or loathe them!

Chillies
Dried chilli flakes or powders are brilliant for pepping up soups, stews and baked beans – one study also suggests they might help with fat-burning and increasing the metabolism.

Chopped fresh chillies are wonderful, of course – you can grow your own or buy a plant and keep it on a sunny windowsill. Be careful, though, as they're truly potent just off the tree: I once had a coughing fit when I sliced one open, from all the oils it released! Try: www.dartmoorchillifarm.com

Chilli sauces and pastes offer a fast and controllable way to add a kick. I live down the road from Chilli Pepper Pete (www.chillipepperpete.com), a shop devoted to every possible use of the fiery fruits. There are *hundreds* of sauces. They do mail order, too.

Chutneys/pickles

I am addicted to all things sweet and sour, including pickles and chutneys. Be mindful of the sugar content, but a small amount, calorie-counted, can give you a much-needed hit of flavour. Spread some very thinly on a slice of bread, add a slice of low-cal cheese and grill for a Fast Day cheese on toast.

Garlic

Low in calories, good for the heart and a little goes a very long way. It's much less potent if you roast it along with other vegetables. Break it into cloves but leave them in their pink skins until they're roasted, then squeeze out as a purée. You can even spread it on a slice of bread if you're brave; it's as unctuous as butter.

Herbs

I don't often use dried herbs but if you like them, they'll liven up grilled or baked meat and fish dishes.

Frozen herbs or bottled herbs in vinegar or oil can work, though I still prefer fresh. The most versatile are flat-leaf parsley, chives and basil. In the summer, I grow my own and often the plants survive to live another day next spring; and in winter I manage to keep pots of supermarket herbs going for quite a while (though I always fail with coriander).

Rocket or young spinach leaves work well both as a salad crop and added to soup or stews to add body and taste.

Horseradish/wasabi

I love the scary-hot tang of wasabi (the green horseradish you get in pre-packed sushi trays or in a tube) even though the tiniest quantity can make your eyes water! The combination of pain and pleasure certainly takes your mind off fasting.

Miso

This Japanese fermented paste comes in jars or tubes and adds a meaty (though it's veggie) flavour to all sorts of dishes. It also works as a very low-cal soup when mixed with boiling water in a mug. You can buy it as powdered sachets ready to make into soup, which may be more convenient to take to work.

Mustard

I love every kind: Dijon, English, American and wholegrain. Even the ones with beer or honey aren't off-limits as long as you check the calories and use sparingly.

Olives/tapenade

A jar of olives in the cupboard is a good Fast Day option, although do check the calories. Tapenade, an olive paste, adds flavour and saltiness.

Salsa

Fresh is best (see the recipes on pages 309–311) but the jarred ones aren't bad. As salsa usually doesn't contain sugar, it's often a better option than tomato ketchup.

Soy sauce

Adds a salty flavour to dressings and stir-fries. I prefer the dark version, which is richer.

Spices

My basics are the ones I keep in the masala dabba, as listed on page 127. I also keep a whole nutmeg for grating, plus a pot of garam masala, which is a lovely warming blend.

Generally, ground spices keep less well than whole, but you can grind your own mix in a pestle and mortar or even a coffee grinder if you want to be really precise about it. I prefer pre-mixed pastes to curry powders for Thai or Indian dishes, though the calories vary greatly, so check the labels.

Sweeteners

I could write a whole book on artificial sweeteners and still not answer all the questions and concerns people have. I think it's a personal choice about whether to use artificial or not. All food additives in developed countries are thoroughly tested before they're approved and that means I am OK with using them if required. Although I have a sweet tooth, I don't add sweeteners to hot drinks, and in dressings I'll use either honey or a sweetener based on Stevia, which is of plant origin. Personally, I don't see much benefit in using agave nectar over honey or even normal sugar, as it is very expensive. It may have less effect on blood sugar but processing can make that advantage disappear.

Vinegars

Cider or wine vinegars can dress salads, as can balsamic, although the latter is more calorific as it's sweet, coming in at between 4 and 16 calories per tablespoon depending on the brand. Vinegar also has health benefits and may improve insulin sensitivity.

Worcestershire sauce

A few drops of sauce adds flavour but if you're a veggie, look for an anchovy-free variety or try mushroom ketchup.

CHAPTER FOUR

Comfort Food

BIG-HEARTED DISHES FOR FLATTER BELLIES

Stews, pasta, pies . . . words that make you feel warm inside. After my first 5:2 winter, one of the coldest on record, I've realised how important comfort food is to staying on track.

Many of us find that the first Fast Days can make you feel colder. Hot drinks help and there are lots of new ideas for those later in this book (see pages 283–287), but a hearty meal that's low in calories will warm you up from the inside out. Many of the dishes in this chapter are great for family meals and are at the higher end of the 500–600 allowance, so they'll work particularly well if you prefer to eat once on a Fast Day. They also tend to lend themselves to batch cooking and freezing if you're cooking for one.

The phrase 'comfort food' sometimes makes us feel guilty, but actually, food *is* a pleasure and a comfort on chilly days. These big-hearted dishes will warm your cockles, without sabotaging your Fast Day. Seriously, what's *not* to love?

RECORD

RECIPES

CLAIRE'S DIET COKE CHICKEN

LEMON AND PORK MEATBALLS WITH
CHUNKY TOMATO SAUCE

BEEF AND ALE STEW

SPAGHETTI BOLOGNESE

SKINNY MINI POPEYE PIES

CRUNCHY BUTTERMILK CHICKEN WITH BALSAMIC
ROASTED TOMATOES AND COURGETTES

BASIL AND LEMON BAKED SALMON EN PAPILLOTE
WITH ROASTED FENNEL

THE BEST VEGETARIAN COTTAGE PIE

ONE-TRAY BAKED COD PROVENÇAL

SKINNY CHICKEN KIEVS

GRILLED MACKEREL WITH ROASTED BEETROOT,
WATERCRESS AND HORSERADISH AND BALSAMIC DRESSING

5:2 Lives

CLAIRE'S SWEET SUCCESS

'My doctor approves of 5:2 - and I'm seeing amazing results.'

Claire Cowking, from Trafford in Manchester, had a very specific reason for trying 5:2. She was diagnosed with type 1 diabetes as a child and has monitored her blood sugar levels – and their effect on her health – ever since.

'I knew that those with type 2 diabetes had marked improvements in health conditions while on 5:2 so I decided to give it a go. I knew it would help with diabetic control and I needed to lose 16kg (35 lb). Diet clubs weren't working and I found normal diets unsustainable.'

Claire, who's 38 and lives with her husband and teenage son and daughter, spoke to her specialists before starting, although she's made herself an expert too. Her body doesn't produce insulin so instead she has to use an insulin pump, which takes a reading of her blood sugar every five minutes. It means she's in a position to see how 5:2 is directly improving insulin sensitivity – in other words, how fast and effectively the insulin gets to work.

And after just a few weeks on her new regime, she was already seeing some very significant results. 'Before I started, I was averaging an intake of 55 units per day. After a month, my five-day average is now (drum roll) 35.5 units per day – a massive reduction!'

Claire explains exactly why the figures are good news: 'It proves that this way of eating increases insulin sensitivity, and so will help you lose weight and reduce cholesterol. I can see the reduction in insulin spikes and improvements in insulin sensitivity in real, tangible measures.'

As well as the obvious health benefits, Claire's also losing around 0.45kg (1 lb) a week, shifting almost a stone so far, and keeping very active. 'I even managed a 16km (10-mile) mountain bike ride in the snow with a lot of uphill climbs, without breaking my fast! And I'm calmer, yet have more energy than before.'

Claire's new regime also has the seal of approval from the doctor who has been treating her since she was eleven. 'He is retiring this year, but he said that with the way I look after my diet, he is confident that I will live a long and healthy life with minimal diabetic complications. He is in favour of the 5:2.'

Of course, anyone with long-term health issues needs to talk to their own specialist before starting 5:2, but Claire is very happy with her doctor's verdict. 'It meant a lot because he doesn't mince his words and will always tell you straight if he doesn't agree with what you're doing!'

Claire's Fast Day Diary

I usually aim for a total of 485 calories, spread out between lunch and supper. For breakfast I drink a black coffee. I try to stick to under 100 calories for lunch, and will usually have some homemade soup. I'll have a mid-afternoon snack of a pot of sugar-free jelly. Dinner will be something like a Bolognese or other tomato-based meal with zero noodles (see page 144). Where possible, I'll use a non-meat alternative, as meat is much higher in calories. I'll have a supper of a boiled egg and a low-calorie hot chocolate.

I like to include soups and broths for lunches and main meals because I can cook them in bulk and freeze individual portions. We are all home at different times so bulk cooking means everyone can have what they want, when they want it.

Feast Day Secrets

I am still calorie counting on Feast Days, and am aiming for a max of 1690 calories, which would give me a 0.2kg (0.5lb) loss per week. BUT I don't stress too deeply and if I go over, it's not a big deal. Using a food diary even on Feast Days means that if I am struggling to lose weight, I have a reference to look back at and see why. Once I've lost the weight I need to, I'll be doing 6:1.

Favourite Foods

I am a big fan of rump steak with the obligatory bottle of red wine! I also love cheese and biscuits as a dessert. I do crave chocolate sometimes, but try to stick to the 80 per cent cocoa ones as they're kinder on my blood sugar levels.

Fast Day Top Tips

- Try to go for as long as possible before you start eating. Once you take that first mouthful of food, your appetite will probably kick in.

- I do sometimes crave sweet things and sugar-free jelly pots at around 3–6 calories per pot are good to satisfy those. Also try liquorice tea, which helps to suppress the appetite.

The Best Thing About 5:2

You're only ever on a 'diet' for one day, then you are free to eat (within reason) what you want without having 'broken the diet' the following day.

CLAIRE'S DIET COKE CHICKEN

Claire says: 'I love Diet Coke. I've read the different opinions about artificial sweeteners, which are especially relevant to me because I'm diabetic, and personally, I am happy they're safe. Usually I drink my DC, but adding it to chicken is great. The sauce is the key to this recipe; it is sweet yet savoury! You can put what you like in it really, it doesn't have to be chicken. Try Quorn, tofu or beef strips.'

Serves 3–4
Calories per portion: 222–167
Preparation time: 10–15 minutes
Cooking time: 25–30 minutes

  1-cal cooking spray
  1 onion, peeled and diced *38 cals*
  1 clove garlic, crushed *4 cals*
  1 carrot, peeled and diced *34 cals*
  1 green pepper, seeded and cut into bite-sized pieces
     30 cals
  300g skinless chicken breasts, fat trimmed and cut into
     bite-sized pieces *495 cals*
  ½ tsp Chinese five spice
  1 tbsp Worcestershire sauce *5 cals*
  200g passata *60 cals*
  330ml can Diet Coke
  salt and pepper

1. Spray a large non-stick saucepan with 1-cal cooking spray and fry the onion over a medium heat for 2–3 minutes to soften. Stir in the garlic and heat for a further minute. Add the carrot and pepper to the pan and soften for 1–2 minutes.

2. Stir in the chicken pieces along with the Chinese five spice and Worcestershire sauce. Cook, stirring, for 3 minutes.

3. Pour in the passata and Diet Coke and bring to the boil. Reduce the heat to a simmer and cook gently for 20 minutes, stirring occasionally so it doesn't stick to the pan. Loosen with a splash of water if necessary to reach the desired consistency. Serve with Cauliflower Rice (see pages 303–304), green veg or a packet of shirataki noodles (see page 323) that have been well rinsed then simmered in salted water for 5 minutes.

Kate says: when Claire posted about Diet Coke chicken in the 5:2 Facebook group, it caused quite a stir. People recommended lots of variations, including diet orange with tomato for a sweet and sour flavour or diet lemon for Chinese lemon chicken. We haven't tested those versions, but if you're feeling ambitious, give them a try. Other suggestions include adding 100g of tinned, drained water chestnuts or bamboo shoots if you like these extra crunchy vegetables: it'll make the dish go further, too.

LEMON AND PORK MEATBALLS WITH CHUNKY TOMATO SAUCE

These herby, lemony meatballs are amazingly low in calories for such a satisfying dish. They make a great family meal; serve with green beans or, if you have some calories to spare, sweet potatoes or mash. If you're dining alone, they will keep in the fridge for up to three days or they freeze really well for up to three months.

Serves 4
Calories per serving: 160, 174 with beans
Preparation time: 25 minutes
Cooking time: 40 minutes

1-cal cooking spray
2 red onions, peeled and finely chopped *76 cals*
2 cloves garlic, finely chopped *8 cals*
75ml white wine *50 cals*
2 x 400g tins chopped tomatoes *144 cals*
generous pinch dried chilli flakes
pinch caster sugar
250g good-quality pork sausages, skin removed *287 cals*
grated zest of 1 lemon *2 cals*
2 tbsp chopped fresh oregano or sage leaves *10 cals*
1 free-range egg yolk, beaten *64 cals*
salt and pepper
200g green beans, to serve (optional) *54 cals*

1. For the sauce, spray a little 1-cal cooking spray in a large non-stick saucepan. Add the onions, season well and fry over a low heat for 4–5 minutes until softened but not coloured. Remove a third of the cooked onion and set aside to cool for the meatballs.

2. Add the garlic to the pan and fry for 2 minutes. Pour in the wine, turn up the heat and allow to bubble for 2–3 minutes. Stir in the tomatoes, chilli and sugar. Bring to the boil, then turn down the heat and simmer for 20–30 minutes until thickened slightly. Add a splash of water if the sauce is too thick.

3. Tip the reserved cooled onion into a large bowl. Add the sausage meat, lemon zest, oregano and egg yolk. Season, then mix until well combined.

4. Preheat the grill to medium-hot. Wet your hands, then shape the mixture into 20 small balls.

5. Place all the meatballs on a lightly greased baking tray and grill for 15–20 minutes, turning, until golden all over and cooked through. Tip the cooked meatballs into the sauce and heat through.

6. Divide the meatballs and sauce between serving plates and accompany with the steamed green beans, if using.

BEEF AND ALE STEW

The honest, no-nonsense name of this dish still conjures up a wintry kitchen with steamed-up windows, an open fire and your favourite music playing. I can't promise the open fire, but if you sort out the music and lay the table, this feel-good stew will do the rest.

Serves 4
Calories per serving: 439
Preparation time: 15 minutes
Cooking time: 1¾ hours

    1-cal cooking spray
    2 onions, peeled and chopped *76 cals*
    2 carrots, peeled and thickly sliced *68 cals*
    2 sticks celery, thickly sliced *12 cals*
    ½ swede, peeled and cut into cubes *36 cals*
    1 leek, thickly sliced *40 cals*
    2 tbsp tomato purée *9 cals*
    700g extra lean diced beef braising steak *1,120 cals*
    4 tbsp plain white flour *204 cals*
    2 sprigs fresh rosemary
    2 fresh bay leaves
    500ml dark ale (use any darker ale or stout) *150 cals*
    250ml fresh beef stock *12 cals*
    2 tsp redcurrant jelly *27 cals*
    salt and pepper

1. Preheat the oven to 180°C/350°F/Gas mark 4. Spray a little 1-cal cooking spray in a large flameproof casserole. Add the onions and fry over a medium heat for about 5 minutes, until softened and lightly browned.

2. Add the other vegetables and cook for 5–8 minutes, until slightly softened. Stir in the tomato purée and cook for 1 minute.

3. Place the beef in a large bowl, season well, add the flour and toss to coat. Add the beef to the pan with the vegetables and stir well. Add the rosemary, bay leaves, ale and stock, stir well and bring to the boil. Cover with a lid and simmer in the oven for about 1½ hours, until the beef and vegetables are tender.

4. To serve, remove the rosemary sprigs and stir in the redcurrant jelly. This is delicious served with steamed green vegetables.

SPAGHETTI BOLOGNESE

What's a chapter about comfort food without a recipe for spaghetti Bolognese? Like many of these heartier dishes, it's quite high in calories, but the wine-enriched sauce is so worth it. Alternatively, this could be the ideal sauce to try with the Courgette Pasta on pages 321–322. The sauce freezes very well. Leave it to cool completely, spoon into a freezer-proof dish and freeze for up to three months. Defrost completely before heating through until piping hot.

Serves 4
Calories per serving: 211 without spaghetti or Parmesan, but with wine; 397 with spaghetti, Parmesan and wine.
Preparation time: 10 minutes
Cooking time: 50 minutes

1-cal cooking spray
1 onion, peeled and finely chopped *38 cals*
2 sticks celery, finely chopped *12 cals*
1 leek or courgette, finely chopped *40 cals*
2 cloves garlic, finely chopped *8 cals*
400g extra-lean minced beef *480 cals*
2 tbsp tomato purée *10–28 cals*
2 carrots, peeled and coarsely grated *68 cals*
150ml red wine or beef stock *90 cals or 8–15 cals for stock*
400g tin chopped tomatoes *72 cals*
1 fresh bay leaf
500ml hot beef stock *25 cals*

200g wholewheat spaghetti *660 cals*

salt and pepper

20g Parmesan cheese, grated (optional) *84 cals*

1. Spray a medium non-stick saucepan with 1-cal cooking spray. Add the onion, celery and leek or courgette, season well and fry over a gentle heat for 2–3 minutes, until softened. Add the garlic and fry for another minute.

2. Add the beef and fry for 5–6 minutes, until golden brown. Add the tomato purée and grated carrots and cook for 2–3 minutes.

3. Pour in the wine (if using), turn up the heat and let the sauce bubble for 3–4 minutes. Then add the tomatoes, bay leaf and stock. Bring to the boil and simmer for 30 minutes, until the sauce has thickened.

4. Cook the spaghetti according to the packet instructions, drain and then divide between serving plates. Top with the Bolognese sauce. If you can 'spare' the calories, a little grated Parmesan is a great extra.

SKINNY MINI POPEYE PIES

Fast Days get easier and easier. But sometimes I miss the kind of crunch you get from toast, a roast potato or a pie. This *definitely* fills the crunchiness gap! With a good helping of creaminess and a huge herb hit into the bargain. Be generous with your handful of parsley, mint or chives.

The filling is based on the spinach and ricotta filling you find in Greek spanakopita pies. Wrapping the filling in pastry just adds calories, and it's hard to avoid soggy filo on the bottoms without loads of fat. So in this recipe you get all the flavour and crunch, without the soggy bottoms. You can either make them in individual ramekins – for mini pies – or in a bigger soufflé dish for a family meal. So pretty and spring-like, no one will realise they're sharing a fast dish!

Serves 4
Calories per serving: 199
Preparation time: 5 minutes
Cooking time: 26 minutes

  100g baby spinach leaves or 110g frozen leaf spinach
    25 cals
  100g low-fat feta cheese, crumbled *180 cals*
  250g ricotta cheese *335 cals*
  handful mixed fresh herbs e.g. parsley, mint, coriander, rocket,
    chives, dill, chopped *5 cals*
  2 eggs, beaten *156 cals*
  4–5 spring onions, finely chopped *6 cals*

grated nutmeg, to taste (lots, in my case)
salt and pepper
1-cal cooking spray
2 sheets filo pastry *88 cals (but check the packet)*

1. Preheat oven to 180°C/350°F/Gas mark 4. Blanch the spinach in boiling water for 45 seconds (or in the microwave for the same time). Drain away as much water as possible, squeeze dry and then chop finely. If you're using frozen spinach, cook and drain thoroughly according to packet instructions. Allow the spinach to cool.

2. Mix the cheeses, cooled spinach, chopped herbs, eggs and spring onions together in a bowl. Grate over the nutmeg then season with a little more salt and pepper than you think it might need. Spoon the mixture into a dish or individual ramekins and cook in the oven for 10 minutes.

3. Take a filo sheet, tear it in half and scrunch it lightly, like tissue paper. Pop it on top of the pie dish so it fills roughly one quarter of the space. Repeat with the other half and then the other sheet of filo. Spray the top with 1-cal cooking spray (use 3 or 4 sprays to give a light covering). If you're using individual ramekins, use half a sheet for each ramekin to cover the filling.

4. Bake for 10–15 minutes until brown (keep an eye on it to make sure it doesn't burn). This is so good served with steamed broccoli or sugar snap peas, and or a fresh tomato salad.

Variations: The filling is also fantastic in grilled peppers. You can use the same crunchy filo idea for other 'pies'; try it with the Mushroom Stroganoff or Chilli con Carne (see pages 246–247 or 125–126). For a 5:2 pie in red and green, make the egg, cheese and onion mix in a bowl, then add 50g spinach (*13 cals*) and a handful of herbs to one half, and a tablespoon of sun-dried tomato purée (*10–15 cals*) and 5 finely chopped black olives (*25 cals*) to the other half, mixing well. Put the red layer into the dish first, then the green layer and cook in the oven as overleaf. The two layers may mix a little but it won't affect the taste!

CRUNCHY BUTTERMILK CHICKEN WITH BALSAMIC ROASTED TOMATOES AND COURGETTES

Another winner when it comes to the crunch of Fast Days. The buttermilk marinade makes the chicked beautifully tender, to contrast with the crispiness of the fabulous crumb, herb and Parmesan cheese coating. It's a winner to serve to non-fasting friends or family members, but easy to reduce the ingredients to serve 1, too. I love any leftover tomatoes on toast on a Feast Day!

Serves 4
Calories per serving: 325
Preparation time: 15 minutes, plus marinating
Cooking time: 20 minutes

4 x 110g skinless chicken breasts, fat trimmed *726 cals*
284ml buttermilk *98 cals*
100g fresh breadcrumbs *268 cals*
zest of 1 lemon
pinch dried chilli flakes
2 tbsp chopped fresh oregano *10 cals*
20g Parmesan cheese, finely grated *84 cals*
1-cal cooking spray
2 courgettes, thickly sliced *68 cals*
2 tsp balsamic vinegar *4–12 cals*
200g cherry tomatoes, on the vine *40 cals*
salt and pepper

1. Place the chicken breasts in a large shallow bowl, pour over the buttermilk and leave to marinate for 2 hours or overnight if time allows.

2. Preheat the grill to medium-high. In a large shallow bowl, mix together the breadcrumbs, lemon zest, chilli flakes, half the oregano and the Parmesan and season with salt and pepper. Remove the chicken from the buttermilk, shake off the excess and then coat in the crumbs. Spray the chicken with 1-cal cooking spray.

3. Place the chicken on a baking tray and grill for 15 minutes, turning half way through, until golden on both sides and cooked through.

4. Meanwhile, preheat the oven to 220°C/425°F/Gas mark 7. Place the courgettes in a shallow ovenproof dish, drizzle with balsamic vinegar and scatter with the rest of the oregano. Season with salt and pepper and spray with 1-cal cooking spray. Bake for 10 minutes, then place the cherry tomatoes on top and bake for 8–10 minutes, until the courgettes are just tender and the tomatoes have softened.

5. Serve a piece of chicken per person and then divide the tomatoes and courgettes between the plates.

BASIL AND LEMON BAKED SALMON EN PAPILLOTE WITH ROASTED FENNEL

Who doesn't love a parcel? Cooking the salmon in a baking-paper parcel helps seal in all the lemon and herb flavours – until you open the package at the table. All together now: happy Fast Day to you, happy Fast Day to you!

Serves 2
Calories per serving: 236
Preparation time: 10 minutes
Cooking time: 30 minutes

> 1 large fennel bulb, core removed and finely sliced *31 cals*
> 200g baby leeks, sliced thickly on the diagonal *44 cals*
> 1-cal cooking spray
> grated zest and juice of ½ lemon *9 cals*
> 2 x 125g salmon fillets, skin removed *350 cals*
> 2 tbsp chopped fresh basil *10 cals*
> 175g cherry tomatoes *27 cals*
> salt and pepper

1. Preheat the oven to 200°C/400°F/Gas mark 6. Arrange the fennel and leek slices in a shallow baking tray and spray with a little 1-cal cooking spray. Season well with salt and pepper and sprinkle the lemon juice over the top. Bake for 10–15 minutes.

2. Cut out two large squares of non-stick baking paper. Divide the cooked fennel and leek between the squares of paper and make a small mound in the middle. Place the salmon fillets on top and spray with a little more

cooking spray. Scatter with the basil and lemon zest and place the cherry tomatoes around the salmon.

3. Wrap up the parcels tightly and bake for 10–12 minutes, until the salmon is just cooked through. To serve, place one parcel on each plate and open them at the table.

THE BEST VEGETARIAN COTTAGE PIE

Comfort food isn't only for meat-eaters. And veggie food isn't only for vegetarians. This has all the flavour to convert carnivores: the super-tasty mash topping and rich filling make it the kind of dish you'll cook over and over again. If you have them, add 15g dried, pre-soaked porcini mushrooms (*39 calories*) to the other mushrooms to add even more savoury, earthy tastes.

Serves 4
Calories per serving: 272
Preparation time: 30 minutes
Cooking time: 1 hour

1-cal cooking spray
1 onion, peeled and finely chopped *38 cals*
2 carrots, peeled and finely chopped *68 cals*
2 sticks celery, finely chopped *12 cals*
2 cloves garlic, finely chopped *8 cals*
200g chestnut mushrooms, sliced *26 cals*
3 sprigs fresh thyme, leaves picked
300g pre-cooked or tinned green or Puy lentils *200 cals*
200g baby spinach leaves, chopped *50 cals*
2 fresh bay leaves
200ml hot vegetable stock *8 cals*
2 tsp mushroom ketchup *15 cals*
salt and pepper

For the topping

650g peeled floury potatoes, chopped into even-sized pieces
  552 cals
2 tbsp half-fat crème fraîche *52 cals*
1 tsp Dijon mustard *5–10 cals*
2 tbsp semi-skimmed milk *14 cals*
1 leek, finely sliced *40 cals*

1. Spray a large non-stick saucepan with 1-cal cooking spray. Add the onion, carrots and celery, season with salt and pepper and fry over a medium heat for 5 minutes. Add a splash of water to help them steam.

2. Stir in the garlic and mushrooms, turn up the heat and cook for about 4 minutes.

3. Add the thyme, bay leaves, lentils and stock and simmer for 3–4 minutes. Stir in the spinach and mushroom ketchup and leave for 2 minutes, until wilted.

4. While the lentils are cooking, tip the potatoes for the topping into a pan of salted water and boil for about 15 minutes until tender. Drain well, then mash with the crème fraîche, mustard and milk, and season well.

5. Steam the leek over a pan of boiling water for 3–4 minutes, until tender and then stir into the mash.

6. Preheat the oven to 200°C/400°F/Gas mark 6. To assemble the pie, spoon the lentil mixture into a 1-litre ovenproof dish and top with the mash. Bake for 30 minutes, until piping hot throughout and the topping is golden brown.

ONE-TRAY BAKED COD PROVENÇAL

Before you read this recipe, take a look at the photo. Don't you want a dose of all that sunny Provençal flavour *right* now? Even better, it's one of the simplest recipes in this book. What are you waiting for?

Serves 2
Calories per serving: 247
Preparation time: 10 minutes
Cooking time: 20 minutes

1 red pepper, seeded and cut into wedges *30 cals*
1 yellow pepper, seeded and cut into wedges *30 cals*
1 courgette, thickly sliced *34 cals*
1 red onion, peeled and sliced *38 cals*
1-cal cooking spray
2 x 150g cod fillets, skin removed *288 cals*
100g cherry tomatoes *20 cals*
30g drained and rinsed pitted black olives *40 cals*
zest and juice of ½ lemon *9 cals*
1 tbsp fresh oregano or thyme leaves *5 cals*
salt and pepper

1. Heat the oven to 200°C/400°F/Gas mark 6. Place the chopped peppers, courgette and onion in a shallow baking dish. Spray with a little 1-cal cooking spray, season well with salt and pepper and roast for 10 minutes.

2. Place the cod fillets on top, season and spray with 1-cal cooking spray. Scatter the tomatoes, olives and lemon zest around the fish, and squeeze

over the lemon juice. Sprinkle with the herbs, season again, and bake for 8–10 minutes, until the cod has just turned a denser white colour (this shows it's cooked). Scatter with the olives and serve immediately.

SKINNY CHICKEN KIEVS

I remember the first time my mum cooked a chicken Kiev – the newest, most sophisticated dinner on the block. The crispy breadcrumbs, the soft chicken and then the sudden release of the garlicky filling: no wonder I asked for them to be a regular dinner. This is our 5:2 version. It is much lower in calories than the regular shop-bought Kievs, without losing any of the herby fabulousness!

Serves 4
Calories per serving: 376
Preparation time: 30 minutes, plus chilling
Cooking time: 30 minutes

2 large cloves garlic, crushed *8 cals*
finely grated zest of ½ lemon and a squeeze of juice *4–5 cals*
2 tbsp finely chopped fresh flat-leaf parsley *10 cals*
1 tbsp finely chopped fresh tarragon or 2 tbsp chopped fresh basil *5–10 cals*
4 tbsp low-fat cream cheese, chilled *88 cals*
4 x 100g skinless chicken breasts, fat trimmed *660 cals*
50g plain white flour, well-seasoned with salt and pepper *168 cals*
2 eggs, beaten *156 cals*
75g Japanese panko breadcrumbs *270 cals*
1 tbsp light olive oil *135 cals*
salt and pepper

1. To make the filling, place the garlic, lemon zest and juice, parsley, tarragon or basil and cream cheese in a small bowl. Season with salt and pepper and beat together.

2. Butterfly the chicken breasts by slicing them part of the way through with a sharp knife to make a pocket. Be careful not to slice all the way through to the other side.

3. Season each flattened chicken breast with salt and pepper. Place a quarter of the filling in the centre of each breast. Roll each breast tightly in cling film and chill for 30 minutes to firm up.

4. Preheat the oven to 200°C/400°F/Gas mark 6. When firm, remove the stuffed chicken breasts from the cling film and roll in the seasoned flour. Shake off the excess, dip in the beaten egg, then roll in the breadcrumbs to coat completely.

5. Heat the oil in an ovenproof frying pan over a medium-low heat. Cook the chicken Kievs on all sides until lightly browned, then transfer to the oven and bake for 20 minutes, until golden and cooked through. Serve immediately. These are great with steamed green beans or broccoli.

GRILLED MACKEREL WITH ROASTED BEETROOT, WATERCRESS AND HORSERADISH AND BALSAMIC DRESSING

This isn't a stew or pie but it still fits my definition of a heart-warming dish because it's so tempting, filling and nutritious. Yes, it's at the higher end of the calorie scale for Fast Day than many dishes, but mackerel, beetroot, watercress and olive oil produce a meal that is rich in vitamins and 'good' fats, so tuck in and feel great.

Serves 1
Calories per serving: 405
Preparation time: 10 minutes
Cooking time: 15–20 minutes

125g cooked beetroot (not in vinegar), drained, cut into
   wedges *54 cals*

½ tbsp balsamic vinegar *3–8 cals*

1-cal cooking spray

1 tsp hot horseradish sauce *10 cals*

1 tsp lemon juice *3 cals*

1 tbsp light olive oil *135 cals*

1 mackerel, filleted and skin scored (approx. 125g) *190 cals*

40g mix of watercress, rocket and spinach leaves *10 cals*

salt and pepper

1. Preheat the oven to 200°C/400°F/gas mark 6. Place the beetroot wedges in a roasting tin, drizzle with the balsamic vinegar and a little 1-cal cooking spray. Season with salt and pepper and roast for about 10–15 minutes.

159

2. Mix together the horseradish, lemon juice and olive oil and season. Add a little water to thin it down if necessary.

3. Preheat the grill to high, season the mackerel fillets and grill for 2 minutes on each side, until golden and just cooked through.

4. Pile the mixed leaves on a plate, top with the beetroot and the grilled mackerel fillet, pour over the dressing and serve.

5:2 Know-How

FAMILY EATING

A common question I'm asked is: 'How do I diet when the rest of my family don't need – or don't want – to join in?'

There are two things to think about here. Firstly, the practical issues surrounding cooking for everyone, and secondly, whether you want your younger children to realise you're 'dieting,' especially as fasting is not something children or teenagers should consider.

Juggling Family Meals and Fast Meals

If you're all eating together, many of the meals in this book will appeal to other family members too. You can easily add potatoes to meat or fish dishes, or rice and other side dishes to curries. By doing this, your family probably won't even notice you're not eating as much as them.

If you're worried about being tempted when you prepare something different for the rest of the family, schedule the dishes that they love and you hate for your Fast Days – that way there's no danger of their leftovers knocking you off track! You could also plan a Fast Day for when you're being the taxi service and they have activities, when you all have different mealtimes anyway.

Another option is to cook something similar but lower in calories for yourself, so no one notices. For example, 5:2

dieter Becca invented her pizza recipe so she could eat it alongside her partner (see pages 238–239). Or you may find that the easiest option is to simply 'save' all your calories for your evening meal together, so you can often stick to exactly what they're having.

In many cases, 5:2 can be easier than a regular full-time calorie-controlled diet because with 5:2, you can eat what your children and partner eat most of the time. And, of course, it gives you much more freedom to enjoy celebrations, birthday parties and holidays (see pages 264–265 for more on this).

To Tell or Not To Tell

We all want to set our children a good example and instil sensible attitudes to eating and food, so you may be concerned about how to explain Fast Days, especially as 5:2 is a relatively new idea. No approach is right for everyone: some of our forum members are very happy telling their older children all about the diet, while others prefer to avoid the subject, by maybe saying that they've already eaten.

The choice of language can help; one mum calls Fast Days her 'cleansing' days and the Feast Days her 'nourishing' days. You can also use 5:2 as a chance to discuss healthier food choices – and the fact that treats are part of a balanced diet. I believe that this plan will help you balance your approach to eating and control your appetite – and that your improved attitude towards food will set a great example to children.

Don't forget, it's not only your children whose reactions may surprise you. Partners can have their own views on this, too, and not always helpful ones. They may not understand the science behind the diet, in which case getting them to read one of the books about this might help. Or they may try to sabotage your Fast Days by offering you cakes or sweets. Sometimes change of any kind – even for the better – makes people uncomfortable, so it may help to explain why this is so important to you, especially from the health perspective.

One of the easiest ways to handle adults – partners or grown-up children – is to recruit them to 'the cause' too. Once they see the difference in your weight or wellbeing, it should be pretty easy to convert them.

CHAPTER FIVE

Salad Days

HOT AND COLD SALADS FOR EVERY SEASON

I started following 5:2 in the summer; salads and Fast Days really do go well together. Fresh leaves, juicy tomatoes and luscious dressings seem to make it so much easier.

But why restrict your salads to summer? We have some more substantial salad dishes here that will give you a taste of the sun even when it's freezing outside. Plus, I've put together a list of great salad combinations, to help you invent one that's tailor made to your own likes and dislikes – I can't be the only one who thinks celery is the work of the devil, can I?

As well as the recipes in this chapter, there are lots of great salad dressings in the 5:2 Extras (see pages 312–315). I have jar after jar stored in the fridge, ready for when I fancy chilling out with nothing fancier than some wild rocket, a few slices of red onion and something saucy on top!

RECIPES

BELINDA'S RAW VEGETABLE SALAD WITH A
ZINGY, SPICY DRESSING

SEARED TUNA STEAK WITH FIVE-BEAN SALAD
AND ROCKET DRESSING

SMOKED CHICKEN AND MANGO SALAD

SPICY VIETNAMESE CHICKEN NOODLE SALAD WITH LIME,
MINT AND CHILLI DRESSING

WARM PUY LENTIL, ROASTED PEPPERS AND SPINACH
SALAD WITH BASIL YOGHURT DRESSING

QUINOA SALAD WITH FETA, AVOCADO, PEAS AND SEEDS
WITH LEMON, HONEY AND HAZELNUT DRESSING

CHARGRILLED VEGETABLE SALAD WITH WHOLEWHEAT
GIANT COUSCOUS AND GOAT'S CHEESE

PANZANELLA

ROASTED BEETROOT, PECAN AND GOAT'S CHEESE SALAD
WITH WATERCRESS AND CHICORY

TRIO OF TWISTED WALDORF SALADS

ASPARAGUS, MON AMOUR

REALLY GRATE SALAD IDEAS

MIX-AND-MATCH SUPERFOOD SALAD BAR

5:2 Lives

BELINDA'S FRENCH ADVENTURE

'Yes, the new lean me is under there!'

Belinda Berry knows that the Mediterranean diet is healthy, but she also knows you can have too much of a good thing. With her husband, Graham, she runs photography courses in South West France, where she also cooks for guests. But the region's sumptuous cheeses and meats come at a price.

'It was the huge Hawaiian shirt that I made for my husband at Christmas that made us realise how big we both were! We knew we had to tackle our weight if we were going to avoid diabetes and other health problems.'

By chance, her husband saw something on television about 5:2 and they decided to do it together, although their three cats and four chickens are not joining them on the plan!

In less than two months, Belinda, who is 62, has lost an impressive 7.7kg (16.7 lbs).

'My aim is to get to a healthy BMI, so I set my target at 55kg (121 lb), which is a loss of 13kg (28.6 lb). I'm well over half way and delighted with my new shape! I have a waist again! I've lost 6cm (2.4 in) from my middle and 7cm (2.8 in) from my hips, which were the real problem areas for me. I'm excited about the prospect of shopping for size 12 clothes instead of size 14. My husband has lost 12.6kg (27.7 lb).'

And the health benefits are showing, too: 'I sleep better and my fitness level is definitely improving, as I am really enjoying my weekly Zumba class now.'

Belinda's Fast Day Diary

I am really enjoying the challenge of creating delicious three-course meals with only 400–500 calories! Breakfast is at about 9 a.m. and is a cup of tea with soya milk and either scrambled egg with smoked trout or lean ham, or porridge with berries. I'll then just have black coffee, herbal tea and water during the day. For dinner, at around 8 p.m., we start with a light vegetable soup and then have fish or lean meat, with loads of vegetables. And we usually finish with a light dessert, like fromage blanc with a little fruit.

Feast Day Secrets

Until I reach my target weight I am sticking to an intake of 1,200 calories on my normal days, but with more freedom at weekends to enjoy a glass of wine and whatever treats I feel like. I now don't *need* to count everything, but I do so I can write up my recipes with accurate calorie counts.

As I am such a foodie, I don't want to exclude anything. I like to make the most of seasonal and local produce and so I visit the local markets and buy what looks great as the basis for my weekly meal plan (which I put on my blog; see page 169).

I've found that my appetite has really reduced. I don't stuff myself like I used to, and will stop when I have had enough. I won't finish a plateful just because it is there.

I've also stopped snacking! I used to love Bombay mix with a glass of wine while preparing dinner, but haven't even thought about it for weeks. I only drink wine at weekends or if we go out, and even then I find that I don't drink as much.

Favourite Foods

My food is something of a melting pot, with influences from Spain, Morocco and the Caribbean, as well as the duck, truffle and prune dishes our region is famous for. And it's all blended with a background of traditional British food and a love of Indian, Middle Eastern and Thai flavours! I'm lucky to have the space to grow a lot of food using organic methods – you just can't buy a tomato that tastes as good as a freshly picked one from the garden.

Fast Day Top Tip

- When I feel the hunger pangs, I think of it as being the moment when my body is warning me that it needs more food and is about to start eating . . . me! It is the beginning of fat-burning time. Yes, the new lean me is under there!

The Best Thing About 5:2

It's helped me to learn that it is OK to be hungry for a while, but best of all is that I really feel that I can lose the excess weight and keep it off. It has also given me the inspiration I needed to get my act together to get my food blog started. It's called *Focus On Flavour, 5:2 Healthy Eating for Life*. That sums it up for me! Check it out at www.focusonflavour.com.

BELINDA'S RAW VEGETABLE SALAD WITH A ZINGY, SPICY DRESSING

Belinda says: 'I think it's good for us to eat lots of raw vegetables, so salads are a big feature in our diet. This salad combines different textures with an Asian-inspired spicy dressing. It is so easy to vary according to the different seasons and works either on its own, or with fish, chicken, tofu or eggs. Other veggies you could use include bean shoots, finely sliced spring onions, raw beetroot strips, courgette ribbons, cauliflower florets or shredded cabbage. If you have well-flavoured food, it is easy to be satisfied with a small amount, which is why I called my blog Focus On Flavour (www.focusonflavour.com).'

Serves 2
Calories per serving: 88 with dressing; 53 without
Preparation time: 15 minutes

handful rocket leaves *5 cals*

50g celeriac, peeled and grated or cut into strips *15 cals*

½ sweet red pepper, seeded and cut into strips *15 cals*

¼ cucumber, sliced diagonally *7 cals*

1 celery stick, sliced diagonally *6 cals*

½ carrot, peeled and sliced into ribbons *17 cals*

25g broccoli, cut into small florets *8 cals*

1 tsp sesame seeds, lightly toasted *32 cals*

fresh Thai basil or coriander leaves, to garnish

For the zingy, spicy dressing

grated zest and juice of ½ lime *10 cals*
6–8 drops sesame oil (less than 1 tsp) *45 cals*
½ tsp Thai fish sauce *2 cals*
½ tsp tamari or light soy sauce *2 cals*
1 tsp sweet chilli dipping sauce *11 cals*

1. Arrange the prepared vegetables in individual piles on a serving platter. Sprinkle with sesame seeds and scatter over the basil or coriander leaves to garnish.

2. Whisk together all the dressing ingredients in a small bowl until combined. Transfer to a dipping bowl and serve alongside the vegetables.

Kate says: I love salads, spices and a sesame flavour, and this is as tasty as it sounds. I replaced the fish sauce with soy to keep it veggie. Next time, I'm going to use the dressing on warm veg, Puy lentils and some grilled light Halloumi for a filling fusion (or should that be confusion?) dinner.

SEARED TUNA STEAK WITH FIVE-BEAN SALAD AND ROCKET DRESSING

This is a fresh and fabulous dish that takes hardly any time to prepare but is bursting with nutritious, tasty ingredients. The avocado oil in the dressing gives a fabulous nutty taste, is rich in vitamin E and has cholesterol-lowering properties, but if you don't have any, you can use light olive oil or olive oil that has been infused with lemon.

Serves 2
Calories per serving: 378
Preparation time: 10 minutes
Cooking time: 5 minutes

2 x 125g fresh tuna steak *340 cals*
1-cal cooking spray
60g wild rocket leaves *15 cals*
grated zest of ½ lemon and a squeeze of juice *4 cals*
1 tbsp avocado oil *135 cals*
½ tsp Dijon mustard *2 cals*
60g fine green beans, trimmed and halved *16 cals*
60g frozen edamame beans, defrosted *78 cals*
200g tinned mixed beans, rinsed and drained *166 cals*
salt and pepper

1. Spray the tuna steaks with a little 1-cal cooking spray, season well with salt and pepper on both sides and sear on a hot griddle for 1–2 minutes on each side. Set aside.

2. Place 40g of the rocket, the lemon zest and juice, the oil, mustard and half a tablespoon of water in a small jug blender. Season well and blend coarsely.

3. Boil the green beans for 2 minutes, add the edamame beans and boil for another minute or so, until just tender. Drain and refresh/submerge in cold water – this stops the cooking process instantly so the veg doesn't go mushy.

4. Mix the tinned beans with the green and edamame beans, and stir through the rest of the rocket. Serve the bean salad with the seared tuna on top, drizzled with a little of the dressing.

SMOKED CHICKEN AND MANGO SALAD

I'm a big fan of mixing sweet and savoury tastes in salads, and this mango and chicken dish is an inspired combination. The sweet, luscious mango and herbs really complement the smoked chicken, while the toasted sesame seeds add texture and a nutty flavour. Perfect for summer lunchboxes, too.

Serves 2
Calories per serving: 237
Preparation time: 15 minutes

finely grated zest and juice of ½ lime *10 cals*
½ red chilli, deseeded and finely chopped *2–4 cals*
2 tsp toasted sesame oil *90 cals*
2 tbsp chopped fresh basil leaves *10 cals*
2 tbsp chopped fresh mint leaves *10 cals*
1 tsp clear honey *20 cals*
1 large Little Gem lettuce, leaves separated *15–25 cals*
1 ripe mango, peeled and chopped (about 200g flesh) *120 cals*
100g smoked chicken, thickly sliced *165 cals*
1 tbsp toasted sesame seeds *32 cals*
salt and pepper

1. To make the dressing, whisk together the lime zest and juice with the chilli, sesame oil, basil, mint and honey, then season well with salt and pepper.

2. Place the lettuce leaves in a large bowl, add the chopped mango and sliced chicken, pour over the dressing and toss well to coat. Sprinkle with sesame seeds and serve.

SPICY VIETNAMESE CHICKEN NOODLE SALAD WITH LIME, MINT AND CHILLI DRESSING

I love Vietnamese food for its mix of fresh flavours, spices and the hint of a French influence. This dressing is unbelievably delicious, and the noodles and chicken make it a very filling dish. It's also a time-saver, as the other portion will keep in the fridge for two days – don't add the dressing until just before serving.

Serves 2
Calories per serving: 338
Preparation time: 15 minutes
Cooking time: 10 minutes

juice of 1 lime *20 cals*

1 tbsp fish sauce *5 cals*

2 tbsp sweet chilli sauce *45–55 cals*

1 tsp sesame oil *45 cals*

1 red chilli, deseeded and finely chopped *4–8 cals*

2 Thai shallots or 1 regular shallot, thinly sliced *14 cals*

100g cooked skinless chicken breast, fat trimmed and shredded *165 cals*

150g thin rice noodles *238 cals*

5cm piece cucumber, deseeded and cut into ribbons with a vegetable peeler *10 cals*

75g bean sprouts *23 cals*

large handful fresh coriander leaves *5 cals*

large handful fresh mint leaves *5 cals*

1 tbsp toasted sesame seeds *96 cals*

1. For the dressing, put the lime juice, fish sauce, sweet chilli sauce and sesame oil into a small pan and bring to the boil slowly. Remove from the heat, stir in the chilli and shallots and leave to cool for 10 minutes. Add the shredded chicken and toss to coat in the dressing.

2. Cook the noodles according to the packet instructions, then drain and refresh in cold water.

3. Tip the noodles into a large bowl and gently mix in the cucumber, bean sprouts, coriander and mint leaves. Add the dressed chicken and toss together. Sprinkle with the toasted sesame seeds before serving.

WARM PUY LENTIL, ROASTED PEPPERS AND SPINACH SALAD WITH BASIL YOGHURT DRESSING

A warm salad like this one is a year-round winner – I love the contrast between the earthy lentils and the intensity of the roasted peppers and onions. Such a satisfying dish!

Serves 2
Calories per serving: 238
Preparation time: 15 minutes
Cooking time: 25 minutes

1 red pepper, seeded and sliced *30 cals*
1 yellow pepper, seeded and sliced *30 cals*
1 orange pepper, seeded and sliced *30 cals*
1 red onion, peeled and sliced into wedges *38 cals*
1-calorie cooking spray
1 tsp balsamic vinegar *2–6 cals*
200g tinned Puy lentils, drained *274 cals*
25g sun-blushed tomatoes, drained and chopped *32 cals*
50g baby spinach leaves, roughly chopped *13 cals*
2 tbsp chopped fresh basil *10 cals*
2 tbsp fat-free natural yoghurt *16 cals*
salt and pepper

1. Preheat the oven to 200°C/400°F/Gas mark 6. Mix together the peppers and onion in a roasting tin. Spray with a little 1-cal cooking spray and season well with salt and pepper. Drizzle with the balsamic vinegar and toss together. Roast for about 20 minutes, turning occasionally.

2. Meanwhile, cook the lentils in a saucepan of water over a low heat until just warmed through.

3. Drain the lentils and tip into a large bowl and add the roasted peppers and onion, the sun-blushed tomatoes and the spinach. Season well and mix together.

4. Whisk together the basil and yoghurt with a little water to thin it slightly. Season and then pour over the salad and mix together.

banana oat muffins
(see page 48)

Vanilla granola pots with berry fruit compote (see page 50)

Hearty Tuscan bean soup
(see page 81)

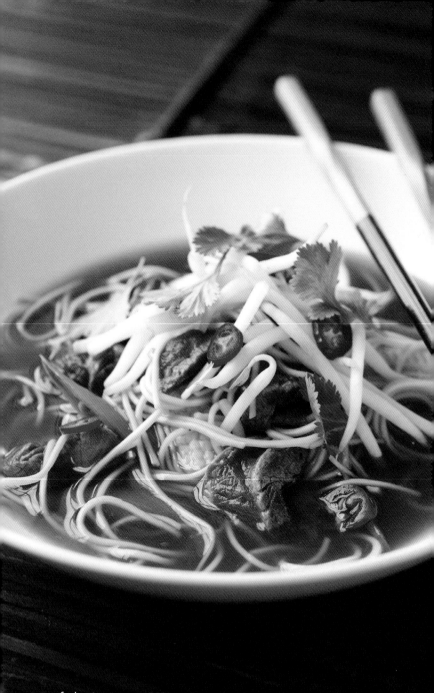

Beef pho (see page 91)

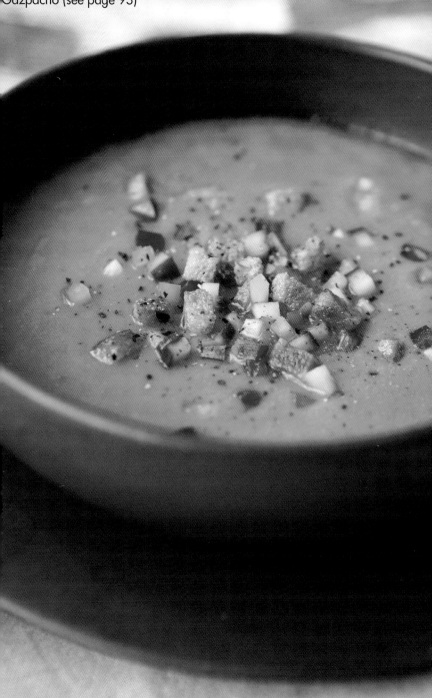

Gazpacho (see page 93)

Lamb kofta in pitta pockets with feta, cucumber salad and minty yoghurt sauce (see page 117)

Spicy Vietnamese chicken noodle
salad with lime, mint and chilli
dressing (see page 175)

Grilled mackerel with roasted beetroot, watercress and horseradish and balsamic dressing (see page 159)

Crunchy buttermilk chicken with balsamic roasted tomatoes and courgettes (see page 149)

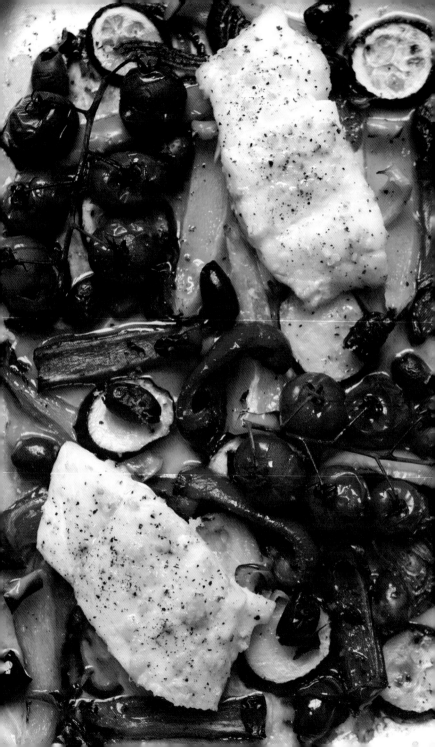

Greek mezze of roasted squash hummus, tzatziki and baba ganoush (see page 240)

❮ One-tray baked cod provençal (see page 155)

Thai prawn skewers with griddled courgette, pea and mint salad (see page 254)

Spicy Mexican bean burgers
(see page 261)

Chargrilled vegetable salad with wholewheat giant couscous and goat's cheese (see page 181)

Cinnamon and vanilla
poached pears (see page 274)

Elderflower jellies with blueberries, raspberries and mint (see page 276)

QUINOA SALAD WITH FETA, AVOCADO AND PEAS WITH LEMON, HONEY AND HAZELNUT DRESSING

This is another favourite of mine. It contains so many foods I love: cheese, avocado, seeds and nuts. Plus, quinoa – a food that has gone from being an obscure Peruvian food, to the trendiest grain (actually a 'pseudo-grain') there is. And no wonder – it's nutty and filling and packed with protein. It's faster to use pre-cooked pouches, but dried is cheaper.

If you want to cut the calorie count, leave out the avocado. This is a single-meal supper that really earns its keep on Fast Day. If you want to cut the calorie count leave out the avocado.

Serves 2
Calories per serving: 426 with avocado; 309 without
Preparation time: 10 minutes
Cooking time: 20 minutes, if cooking the quinoa

125g red and white cooked quinoa *252 cals* or 60g
   uncooked *220 cals*
2 Little Gem lettuces, leaves separated *25–30 cals*
30g low-fat feta cheese, crumbled *54 cals*
1 avocado (about 150g), cut into cubes *235–285 cals*
50g frozen peas, defrosted *25 cals*
20g toasted hazelnuts, chopped *134 cals*
1 tbsp hazelnut oil *134 cals*
2 tsp lemon juice *5 cals*
1 tsp clear honey *20 cals*
salt and pepper

1. If you're using uncooked quinoa, boil it in 120ml water for 20 minutes or until the water has been absorbed and the grains are tender. Set aside and allow to cool.

2. Arrange the lettuces leaves over a large platter and place the quinoa on top of the leaves.

3. Scatter over the feta, avocado, peas and hazelnuts.

4. Whisk together the hazelnut oil, lemon juice and honey, and season well with salt and pepper. Drizzle over the salad just before serving.

CHARGRILLED VEGETABLE SALAD WITH WHOLEWHEAT GIANT COUSCOUS AND GOAT'S CHEESE

Chargrilling veggies gives them a much more intense flavour, and this salad is great for winter as well as summer. The idea of 'giant' couscous always makes me smile . . . but it has a really satisfying texture to accompany the chunky veg.

This salad serves four because we're using a variety of vegtables to add gorgeous, summery colours. But it keeps in the fridge for three days and makes a perfect packed lunch.

Serves 4
Calories per serving: 249 with goat's cheese; 222 without
Preparation time: 15 minutes
Cooking time: 20 minutes

1 red pepper, seeded and cut into wedges *30 cals*

1 orange pepper, seeded and cut into wedges *30 cals*

200g baby leeks *44 cals*

1 courgette, thickly sliced *34 cals*

1-cal cooking spray

1 red onion, peeled and cut into wedges *38 cals*

200g wholewheat giant couscous *666 cals*

400ml hot vegetable stock or water *12–20 cals*

2 tsp harissa paste *14 cals*

finely grated zest of 1 orange and a squeeze of juice *5 cals*

3 tbsp chopped fresh basil *15 cals*

40g goat's cheese, crumbled (optional) *108 cals*

salt and pepper

1. Spray all the vegetables with 1-cal cooking spray and season well with salt and pepper. Heat a griddle pan until smoking hot and griddle the vegetables in batches until nicely charred. Set aside and keep warm while you cook all the batches.

2. Meanwhile, boil the couscous in the vegetable stock or water for 8 minutes, until tender. Top up with water as it is cooking, if necessary. Drain and refresh in cold water.

3. Stir the harissa paste into the couscous and add the orange zest and a squeeze of juice. Stir in the chopped basil. Combine with the chargrilled vegetables and goat's cheese if using, and mix gently.

PANZANELLA

Yum! Bread salad might not sound very promising, but the secret to this is the dressing and the extras. I love it (although I usually leave out the anchovies, as they're too strong for me). You can keep the salad and bread in the fridge for up to three days – the flavours will improve – but keep the bread separately in an airtight container until shortly before serving. For a more substantial meal, you could serve this with salmon or chicken.

Serves 4
Calories per serving: 154 with anchovies; 148 without
Preparation time: 20 minutes, plus chilling
Cooking time: 8 minutes

- 75g country-style granary bread (about 2 days' old), torn into chunks *138 cals*
- 1-cal cooking spray
- 10g Parmesan cheese, freshly grated *42 cals*
- ½ cucumber, roughly chopped *15 cals*
- 3 very ripe tomatoes, roughly chopped (ideally different colours and varieties) *60 cals*
- 50g cherry tomatoes, halved (ideally yellow, orange and red ones if available) *10 cals*
- 1 tbsp extra virgin olive oil *135 cals*
- 2 tsp red wine vinegar *2–5 cals*
- 1 tbsp capers, rinsed and drained *5 cals*
- 1 tsp caster sugar *15 cals*
- 75g drained and rinsed pitted Kalamata olives *158 cals*

4 anchovies, drained and chopped (optional) *26 cals*
2 tbsp chopped fresh basil leaves *10 cals*
salt and pepper

1. Preheat the oven to 200°C/400°F/Gas mark 6. Place the torn bread on a baking sheet, spray with a little 1-cal cooking spray, scatter with the Parmesan and season with salt and pepper. Bake for 6–8 minutes or until golden brown and crisp. Remove from the oven and set aside.

2. Place the cucumber and chopped tomatoes in a large bowl. Whisk together the oil, vinegar, capers, sugar and a little salt and pepper. Pour over the cucumber and tomatoes.

3. Add the olives and anchovies, if using. Stir well and then cover with cling film. Leave in the fridge for an hour or so for the flavours to infuse and develop.

4. About 10 minutes before serving, add the croûtons and basil and mix well to combine.

ROASTED BEETROOT, PECAN AND GOAT'S CHEESE SALAD WITH WATERCRESS AND CHICORY

I've already bored you with my beetroot obsession (see page 75), so now I'll share my passion for pecans! They rock. Oh, and watercress rocks, too, with its high levels of vitamin C and other nutrients. This is the salad of my dreams, and that's official.

Serves 2
Calories per serving: 329
Preparation time: 15 minutes
Cooking time: 20 minutes

125g cooked beetroot (not in vinegar), cut into wedges *54 cals*
2 tsp balsamic vinegar *4–10 cals*
1 tbsp hazelnut or walnut oil *135 cals*
100g goat's cheese, with rind, sliced into 6 rounds
   270–330 cals
1-cal cooking spray
2 sprigs fresh thyme, leaves picked
25g pecan nuts *175 cals*
1 head red or white chicory, leaves separated *9 cals*
40g watercress *11 cals*
salt and pepper

1. Preheat the oven to 180°C/350°F/Gas mark 4. Place the beetroot wedges in a shallow roasting tray. Drizzle half of the balsamic vinegar over the beetroot and spray with 1-cal cooking spray, season with salt and pepper and roast for about 10–15 minutes, until the beetroot is slightly caramelised. Remove from the oven and set aside.

2. For the dressing, whisk together the rest of the vinegar with the oil. Season, then set aside.

3. Preheat the grill to medium. Place the rounds of sliced goat's cheese on a lightly greased baking tray, scatter with the thyme leaves, season and grill for 5 minutes.

4. Add the pecan nuts to the tray and grill for another 1–2 minutes, until the cheese starts to melt and turn golden round the edges and the nuts are turning brown.

5. Divide the chicory and watercress between serving plates and top with the roasted beetroot and pecan nuts.

6. Using a palette knife or fish slice, lift the cheese slices from the tray and transfer to the plates. Drizzle with the dressing and serve immediately.

TRIO OF TWISTED WALDORF SALADS

The traditional Waldorf salad was invented at the luxury New York hotel of the same name in the 1890s. I love a salad that combines fruit, veg and a crunch. Fruit can be an unwise choice when fasting, because it raises blood sugar rapidly, but in this salad it's combined with foods that take longer to digest so it won't have such a dramatic effect. Here are three variations on the Waldorf to make you feel you're in five-star fasting heaven. Each makes enough for two servings, and the first two recipes will keep overnight in the fridge.

Almost Traditional Waldorf

Serves 2
Calories per serving: 125
Preparation time: 10 minutes

1 small, flavourful apple e.g. Cox's Orange Pippin, cored and
    cut into 1cm slices *40–50 cals*
1 large stick celery, sliced *8 cals*
20g walnut halves (if you like, dry-fry them in a small saucepan
    until they smell toasted – remove from heat the instant they
    toast or else they'll burn!), broken into pieces *138 cals*
10 seedless red grapes, halved *34 cals*
Crunchy 'cup-like' lettuce leaves, e.g. ½ Little Gem heart, cut
    into bite-sized pieces *7–9 cals*

For the yoghurt dressing (or use the Creamy Herb dressing on page 313)

2 tbsp fat-free Greek yoghurt *16 cals*
1 tsp cider vinegar *1 cal*
¼ tsp clear honey or pinch sweetener *5 cals*
salt and pepper

1. Combine the fruit, celery and nuts in a large bowl.

2. Make the dressing by putting the ingredients in a jam jar. Screw on the lid and shake well to mix. Alternatively, whisk the ingredients together in a small bowl, until combined and smooth.

3. Add the dressing to the bowl and toss together to coat the salad.

The Pear and Pecan Waldorf

Serves 2
Calories per serving: 138 (plus the dressing calories)
Preparation time: 10 minutes

1 small, ripe (but not mushy) pear, cored and cut into 1cm slices or wedges *45–50 cals*
½ fennel bulb, very thinly sliced, reserving any fennel tops to garnish *31 cals*
20g pecans, dry-fried as for the walnuts in the first recipe, chopped *140 cals*
4 crunchy lettuce leaves, e.g. romaine or Little Gem, cut into bite-sized pieces *5–10 cals*

30g low-fat feta cheese *54 cals*

salt and pepper

For the dressing

1 x portion West Country dressing (see page 314) or the
yoghurt dressing, above

1. Combine all the salad ingredients in a bowl and crumble over the cheese.

2. Mix in the dressing and toss lightly to coat the salad.

Fragrant Orange Waldorf

Serves 2
Calories per serving: 176
Preparation time: 10 minutes

2 ripe oranges *140 cals*

4–5 large radishes, very thinly sliced into circles *5 cals*

10 black olives, pitted and halved *50 cals*

1 tbsp pine nuts, dry-fried as for the first recipe (or shelled
pistachio nuts, *89 cals*) *104 cals*

large handful rocket or watercress leaves *5 cals*

For the dressing

orange juice (from segmenting the oranges for the salad, see
method)

2 tsp lemon juice *2–8 cals*

orange blossom water

1 tsp olive oil *45 cals*

salt and pepper

1. Segment the oranges for the salad using a sharp knife, reserving the juice for the dressing. This will leave you with lush, pith-free pieces. (There are instructions and videos online showing how to do this, but you basically need to cut across the top and bottom of the unpeeled orange. Place the orange on a board and cut away the peel using downward strokes. Cut away any remaining white pith, then slice between the membranes of the orange so you end up with segments.) Pour the juice off the chopping board into a jam jar and squeeze out the juice from the remaining bits of orange and add to the jar.

2. To make the dressing, add the lemon juice, orange blossom water (use just a few drops at a time as it is very potent) and oil to the orange juice. Put the lid on the jar and give it a good shake (alternatively, whisk together the ingredients in a bowl). Taste, and adjust the flavours depending on how much juice came from the oranges. Season, to taste, with salt and pepper.

3. Arrange the orange segments, radishes, olives and pine nuts on a plate. Pour over most of the dressing. Scatter the leaves on top and drizzle with the rest of the dressing.

ASPARAGUS, MON AMOUR

If I had to choose a favourite vegetable, it would probably be asparagus. I love it best drizzled with melted butter, but on a Fast Day it still works brilliantly served with a wedge of lemon and plenty of salt and pepper, or dipped into a poached egg. Plus, asparagus is low in calories and contains high levels of iron, calcium, potassium and vitamins A and C. They have a place in my heart, but there's no place in my tiny kitchen for an asparagus kettle so I boil (with a foil hat to protect the tender tips), steam, or microwave them. You can also add flavour by cooking for a little less time and then griddling in a hot grill pan. Below are some suggestions for other things to eat with asparagus.

Serves 1
Calories per serving: 66
Preparation time: 3 minutes
Cooking time: 7 minutes

  1 small bunch asparagus, about 230g *62 cals*
  zest of ½ lemon and squeeze of lemon juice *4 cals*
  sea salt and pepper

1. Rinse the asparagus and then cut away the woody stems from the bottoms. (The very thin asparagus spears hardly need any trimming at all.)

2. Half-fill a medium saucepan with water and bring to the boil. Form a 'hat' for the asparagus by wrapping foil around them in a cone shape, with the tips at the top and thicker stems at the bottom. Stand the foil cone

in the bottom of the pan and cook for 4–7 minutes depending on the thickness of the stems. (Or you can steam the asparagus in a steamer or microwave them after rinsing (leave a little water on the stalks to stop them drying out) in a shallow dish for 2–4 minutes, until they're tender but not floppy!

3. Serve with a squeeze of lemon juice and some salt and pepper.

Other lovely things to eat with asparagus

15g crumbled low-fat feta cheese (*27 cals*) with a few chilli flakes and chopped fresh parsley or chives.

1 slice crispy Parma ham (see the Hearty Tuscan Italian Bean Soup on page 81) (*31 cals*) and 30g fresh or frozen broad beans (*25 cals*) cooked in the same water as the asparagus.

Butter or Hollandaise sauce! On a Feast Day . . .

POACHING AN EGG

Poaching an egg can be hard to get right. I now use Poach Pods, which are like little green lily pads that you break an egg into and then float in a saucepan of simmering water until the eggs are cooked, which takes 5–6 minutes. However, here's a podless way to do it, which also mean you will get a runnier yolk – extra good for dipping!

Calories per egg: 78
Cooking time: 3 minutes

> 1 egg *78 cals*
> splash vinegar (chip-shop style, not balsamic)

1. Bring a medium saucepan of water to the boil over a medium heat. Add the vinegar as it begins to boil.

2. Break your egg into a small bowl or cup.

3. Create a whirlpool in the water with a fork or whisk and, with your other hand, slip the egg into the middle of the pan as gently as possible.

4. Turn down the heat and set a timer for 3 minutes. Check the white is set before removing from the pan, then use a slotted spoon to transfer the egg to some kitchen paper to absorb the excess water.

Really GRATE Salad Ideas

Forgive the pun, but I've made friends with my food processor's grating disc since starting 5:2 – it's the easiest way to make a lovely grated salad. A box grater will do the job, too, and, once you've dismantled the processor and washed it up, it will probably take about the same amount of time! Every food processor has its quirks, so you may need a few attempts to get perfect grated veg. Shred with the slicing disk or a mandolin if you prefer a chunkier texture.

Use any of the dressings from pages 313–315 to serve with your grated salad, and choose a couple of ingredients from the list of extras to add some variation. Experiment with different combinations and when you have a winner, name your salad after yourself, someone you love or your first pet, and enjoy!

Good veggies to grate	Good things to add
Cabbage Use red or white, or a combination of the two. The slicing disk works well if you want the cabbage shredded rather than finely chopped.	• Creamy dressings (page 313) and a sliced onion make a rather tasty coleslaw • Or add the Nutty Asian Dressing (page 315) or a finely chopped chilli and some soy sauce mixed with a little clear honey • 1 tsp raisins (14 cals) or half a grated apple, plus 1 tsp poppy seeds (28 cals)

Carrots Carrots are one of the few veggies I always try to buy organic as I think they taste better. Top and tail and wash well before grating.	• Lemon juice or balsamic vinegar • 1 tsp toasted sunflower seeds (30 cals) or poppy seeds (28 cals) • 1 tsp raisins (14 cals) • Orange segments (½ orange/35 cals) or a little freshly squeezed orange juice • Whole cumin seeds (dry-fried) (1 tsp/5 cals)
Cucumbers and courgettes The wateriness of cucumbers and courgettes means you will have to squeeze the excess water out after grating and before dressing. Use kitchen paper or a colander. Try yellow and green courgettes for a colourful grated salad.	• Both cucumbers and courgettes benefit from strong flavours; sea salt and fresh grated pepper is a good start • The juice of half a lime (10 cals) or 1 tsp rice vinegar • 1 tsp sesame seeds (32 cals) (dry-fried) with 1 finely chopped red chilli (3–6 cals) • Chopped peanuts (10g/56 cals)

Mix-and-Match Superfood Salad Bar

I'm not sure about the word 'superfood'. It seems a bit *foodist* to elevate some ingredients to that status, especially when scientific developments mean today's hero might be tomorrow's villain. Soya products, for example, were top of the superfood pops for ages, but now it's recognised they're not for everyone due to allergies.

Even so, there is some produce that punches above its weight, nutritionally speaking, so I've put together a guide to help you mix and match combinations that will taste good in a salad *and* give your body a super-serving of vitamins and minerals.

Almonds

Why so super?

High in minerals, mono-saturated fat.

Serving size/approx. calories per serving

1 tbsp flaked almonds/*94.5 cals*

Suggestions

Toasted flaked almonds make a great topping for salads. And whole almonds are a satisfying snack, too, though don't eat many as all nuts are high calorie.

Beetroot

Why so super?

High levels of nitrates that can reduce blood pressure and improve stamina.

Serving size/approx. calories per serving

100g/*43 cals*

1 medium beetroot/*35 cals*

Suggestions

Simply sliced or grated in a salad. Beetroot marries well with fruits and chilli flavours, as well as cumin seeds.

Berries

Why so super?
High in antioxidants, vitamin C and other phytochemicals.

Serving size/approx. calories per serving
100g/*30–60 cals*

Suggestions
Surprisingly good in salad, especially blueberries, dried acais or cranberries (watch for the higher calorie count for dried fruits) or sliced strawberries.

Broccoli

Why so super?
High in vitamin A and isothiocyanates, believed to help fight some forms of cancer.

Serving size/approx. calories per serving
100g/*32 cals*

Suggestions
Great raw and sliced thinly in any salad. Or blanch whole tenderstems and serve with grains and feta or roast squash.

Oily fish

Why so super?
High on omega 3 fats, with potential cardiovascular benefits.

Serving size/approx. calories per serving
100g raw mackerel or salmon/*about 160 cals*

Suggestions

Great as the main event in a salad, mackerel, tuna, sardines and salmon work well with most leaf salads.

Pomegranates

Why so super?

Another fruit high in vitamins and antioxidants.

Serving size/approx. calories per serving

25g/20.5 cals

Suggestions

The seeds look pretty on anything, including dips and salads or in a salsa.

Pulses

Why so super?

High in protein, B vitamins and fibre.

Serving size/approx. calories per serving

100g tinned Puy lentils/*118 cals*
30g hummus/*80 cals*

Suggestions

Hummus is a great way to eat chickpeas. Puy lentils in a salad are earthy and delicious and come tinned or in sachets that don't need cooking.

Pumpkin/squash

Why so super?

High in beta-carotene (the clue is in the vivid colour) and high in vitamins and minerals.

Serving size/approx. calories per serving

100g pumpkin/*20 cals*

100g squash/*40 cals*

Suggestions

Chunks or slices of roasted butternut squash work well in a salad with one or the creamier dressings (see page 313) or some lower-fat cheese like feta.

Quinoa

Why so super?

High in protein, vitamins and minerals.

Serving size/approx. calories per serving

25g dry/*91 cals*

Suggestions

See our salad recipe on pages 179–180 – adapt with other superfoods.

Seeds

Why so super?

High in minerals, omega 3 and 6, and cholesterol-lowering phytosterols.

Serving size/approx. calories per serving

1 tsp (5g)/*30 cals*

Suggestions

Sesame, pumpkin or sunflower seeds add crunch to a salad. Dry-fry to bring out more flavour.

Tangerines

Why so super?

Higher in vitamin C and fibre than many citrus fruits, and research is underway into other benefits including possible cholesterol reducing compounds.

Serving size/approx. calories per serving

1 tangerine/ *40 cals*

Suggestions

Easy to segment and serve with sharper salad flavours and the balsamic or other strong dressings.

Tomatoes

Why so super?

High in vitamins and beta-carotene, plus lycopene, which may fight cell damage and cancer.

Serving size/approx. calories per serving

5 cherry tomatoes/ *20 cals*

Suggestions

Great just as they are. Cooking makes the lycopene more concentrated and available to the body. Try roasting cherry tomatoes or serving cold ratatouille as a dense salad.

Turkey

Why so super?

Great source of lean protein and minerals.

Serving size/approx. calories per serving

100g/ *155 cals*

Suggestions

Use in sandwiches or salads, in place of chicken, with a dressing to counteract any dryness.

Watercress

Why so super?
Very high in vitamin C, with possible cancer-fighting properties.

Serving size/approx. calories per serving
1 handful/ *3 cals*

Suggestions
Peppery watercress peps up most salads or makes a great summery soup

Yoghurt

Why so super?
Live yoghurt contains probiotics that aid digestion. High in calcium.

Serving size/approx. calories per serving
Full-fat Greek yoghurt/100ml *130 cals*
Fat-free Greek yoghurt/100ml *55 cals*

Suggestions
Dressings and dips help you get your ration.

5:2 Know-How:

VEG BOX MAGIC

Veg boxes – a carton of seasonal produce from local farmers delivered to your door every week – have grown in popularity and come down in price. They're now a great way to get your five-a-day and you can often ask not to be sent the foods you hate or don't want to use. I always ask them to leave out celery because I hate the stuff! Or you may want to avoid potatoes because you won't use them on Fast Days.

The boxes are always fun to open and offer a great framework for your 5:2 week. They're also a good option if you don't have time or space to grow your own. Here are some ideas for using a typical box for your Fast and Feast Days. I'm not suggesting you go 100 per cent veggie, although you could consider making all your meals vegetable-based on one of your two Fast Days to encourage you to experiment with new dishes and produce.

Spring/Summer Veg Box Typical Contents

Aubergines
Fast Day 1 main: mezze including aubergine Baba Ganoush (see page 242)
Fast Day 2 side: serve griddled with Creamy Herb Dressing (see page 313) and pomegranate seeds

Broccoli

Fast Day 1 main: Thai Green Curry (see pages 108–109)

Fast Day 2 side: steam florets for 6–9 minutes and serve with Nutty Asian Dressing (see page 315)

Cucumber

Fast Day 1 main: Belinda's Raw Vegetable Salad (see page 170)

Fast Day 2 side: Lamb Kofta with Cucumber Salad (see page 116)

Leeks

Fast Day 1 main: Best Vegetarian Cottage Pie (see pages 153–154)

Fast Day 2 soup: Spring Vegetable and Pesto Minestrone (see pages 83–84)

Little Gem Lettuces

Fast Day 1 main: Quinoa Salad with Feta (see pages 179–180)

Fast Day 2 snack: Avocado Little Gem 'Open Sandwiches' (see pages 220–221)

Red Peppers

Fast Day 1 main: Warm Puy Lentil, Roasted Peppers and Spinach Salad (see pages 177–178)

Fast Day 2 soup: Gazpacho (see pages 93–94)

Vine Tomatoes

Fast Day 1 main: Panzanella (see pages 183–184)

Fast Day 2 side: Grilled Balsamic Tomatoes (from Crunchy Buttermilk Chicken, see pages 149–150)

Autumn/Winter Veg Box Typical Contents

Beetroot

Fast Day 1 main: Roasted Beetroot, Pecan and Goat's Cheese Salad with Watercress and Chicory (see pages 185–186)

Fast Day 2 soup: Ruby Soup (see pages 75–77)

Butternut Squash

Fast Day 1 soup: Kirsty's Butternut and Sweet Potato Soup (see pages 73–74)

Fast Day 2 side: Roasted Squash Hummus (see page 240)

Carrots

Fast Day 1 main: Hearty Tuscan Bean Soup (see pages 81–82)

Fast Day 2 side: Grated Carrot Salad (see page 195)

Cauliflower

Fast Day 1 main: Vegetable Biryani (see pages 254–255)

Fast Day 2 side: Cauliflower Rice with Skinny Chilli con Carne (see pages 303–304 and 125–126)

Courgettes

Fast Day 1 main: Thai Prawn Skewers with Griddled Courgette, Pea and Mint Salad (see pages 254–255)

Fast Day 2 side: Courgette Pasta (see pages 321–322)

Pak Choi
Fast Day 1 main: Sticky Indonesian Pork Stir-Fry (see pages 123–124)
Fast Day 2 soup: Udon Noodle and Miso Soup (see pages 89–90)

Portobello Mushrooms
Fast Day 1 main: Portobello Mushroom Rarebit (see pages 56–58)
Fast Day 2 soup: Brandied Mushroom Soup (see pages 78–80)

Growing Your Own, the Easiest Way Possible

Even if you don't have a garden or space for a window box, you can still sprout your own seeds in a jam jar or sprouting tray, as you don't even need any compost. Like mustard and cress, but turbo-charged for the twenty-first century!

Seeds are easy to grow and much cheaper than buying fancy 'micro leaves' from supermarkets. Plus, they're very nutritious and add great flavour to salads. I like broccoli and alfalfa. It's very simple but slightly fiddly to explain here, so there are lots of online guides to sprouting – you'll be surprised at the variety you can harvest!

CHAPTER SIX

5:2 To Go

PACKED LUNCHES (AND PICNICS!)

Work can *really* sabotage your Fast Days with people bringing in cakes or trying to talk you into 'just one biscuit' at elevenses. I hear school staffrooms are the worst, with nurses' stations coming a close second.

One solution is to get your colleagues on board. It's already happening in some workplaces, with colleagues on a night shift or in the same office bringing 5:2 foods in on the same days.

Taking your meal to work with you helps you avoid the temptation of the canteen or vending machine. In this chapter are some of my top picks, but remember to check out the other chapters for soups, hot dishes and salads that can also work well when you're on the go.

And if the sun shines, why not take an avocado wrap or prawn roll to the beach or the park for a 5:2 picnic? Everything tastes so much nicer eaten out of doors.

RECIDES

RECIPES

FIONA'S ASIAN CHICKEN LETTUCE WRAPS

SWEET POTATO FALAFEL POCKETS

VIETNAMESE PRAWN SUMMER ROLLS

TUNA NIÇOISE WRAPS

AVOCADO WRAPS OR LITTLE GEM 'OPEN SANDWICHES'

GRANOLA SQUARES

BERRY BLAST SMOOTHIE

STICKY BANANA AND DATE BREAD

THE 5:2 LUNCHBOX

5:2 Lives

FOODIE FIONA'S PERFECT FIT

'I eat out at least twice a week, sometimes more, but with 5:2 I can still lose weight.'

Every food lover dreams of reviewing restaurants for a living, but for London-based Fiona Maclean, a freelance writer and marketing consultant, the pleasures of five-course meals at the hottest new eateries in town were starting to be outweighed by the pain of stepping on the scales. In September 2012, Fiona, aged 52, realised that she had to face up to what restaurant reviewing was doing to her body.

'I do a lot of restaurant reviews and eat out far too much. I'm really conscious that I could have health problems in the future, as my Dad and Uncle both had heart attacks and my Mum had diabetes. And I'd put on a lot of weight! I'm only 156cm (5ft 1 in), and weighed 72kg (159 lb) when I started 5:2 (ouch!).'

Fiona soon found that the flexibility of 5:2 and the freedom to eat out was the perfect fit for her. After six months, she'd lost 9kg (20 lb) and is now tantalisingly close to her goal.

'I really want to get into the healthy weight zone, which, for me, is a maximum of 60kg (132 lb). I have hypothyroidism, so that makes losing weight even harder, but currently I am 63kg (139 lb) – nearly there!'

The health improvements have also been striking: 'I feel much better. My feet and ankles were getting swollen and uncomfortable but not anymore. I haven't had a cold all winter and I generally have more energy after a Fast Day. I also don't ache as much (that's connected with the thyroid problem) and my asthma seems better.'

Food-lover Fiona has also found the perfect place to document her 5:2 experiences – and her fantastic recipes – on her blog, www.london-unattached.com.

Fiona's Fast Day Diary

On waking at around 7.30 a.m., I'll have a matcha tea. I generally don't need to eat anything in the morning, but if I'm feeling hungry, I'll have a small portion of fat-free Greek yoghurt with half a teaspoon of clear honey.

I eat lunch at 1 p.m. when I'll have homemade veggie soup – spinach, tomato and lentil, broccoli or celeriac and leek. Supper is at 7 p.m., and I'll usually have a vegetable stir-fry made with shirataki noodles and chicken or prawns, or a vegetable curry.

I drink green tea in the mornings and coffee with milk in the afternoons – I allow for some skimmed milk in my calories on a Fast Day.

Feast Day Secrets

I eat out at least twice a week, and sometimes more. For the most part, review meals are intense affairs with five or more courses not being unusual. I love good food and wine but since starting 5:2, I've found that I can't always eat as much as I used to, and generally prefer to have petit fours to a full dessert, for example. I'm also choosing lighter dishes from the menu – fish or chicken rather than steak – and avoiding some of the dishes with really rich cream-based sauces.

When I'm at home, I generally eat quite healthy food anyway, but sometimes this is coloured by having an ingredient to write about or food to review.

Favourite Foods

Steak, which I really shouldn't eat! Venison and game are a good substitute for the steak for me. I also love fresh, well-cooked vegetables. And afternoon tea!

Fast Day Tip

• I find miso soup or Japanese rice crackers are excellent to ward off hunger pangs.

The Best Thing About 5:2

5:2 lets me lead a normal (for me) lifestyle when it isn't a Fast Day and still seems to work! If I have a really OTT week then I don't lose weight, but as long as I do two Fast Days, I seem to stay the same weight. If I am not out every possible night, then I seem to be losing weight steadily. And, having had the thyroid problem for a few years, that is quite remarkable in its own right.

FIONA'S ASIAN CHICKEN LETTUCE WRAPS

Fiona says: 'For me, one of the challenges of a 5:2 Fast Day menu is how to eat well without including a large portion of rice or potatoes, particularly in winter when I yearn for warm food rather than salads. My favourite local Chinese restaurant serves Hunan, Szechuan and Taiwanese food and one of my favourite dishes is called 'nest of imperial jewels' – chopped prawns with mustard greens, served in an iceberg lettuce leaf. I decided to make my own version for a 5:2 Fast Day. It was absolutely delicious! It's spicy though, so if you prefer a milder flavour use half a chilli rather than a whole one, but chilli and ginger are said to help your metabolism.'

Serves 1
Calories per serving: 319
Preparation time: 25 minutes, plus marinating
Cooking time: 6 minutes

- 1 tbsp soy sauce *3 cals*
- ½ tbsp oyster sauce *7 cals*
- ½ tbsp mirin (a kind of rice wine) *20 cals*
- 1 red chilli, deseeded and finely sliced *4–8 cals*
- 1 clove garlic, crushed or finely chopped *4 cals*
- ½ tsp cornflour *18 cals*
- 1 x 100g skinless chicken breast, fat trimmed and sliced into matchstick-sized strips along the grain *165 cals*
- 1 tsp sesame oil (to cut calories, you can use 1-cal cooking spray instead) *45 cals*

1 spring onion, trimmed and sliced into 0.5cm pieces *2 cals*

1 small carrot, peeled and finely diced *25 cals*

1 stick celery, finely diced *6 cals*

½ small onion, peeled and finely chopped (or use a second
spring onion, finely diced) *15 cals*

2cm piece fresh root ginger, peeled and grated or finely
chopped *2 cals*

salt and pepper

3 iceberg lettuce leaves, to serve *3 cals*

fresh coriander leaves, to garnish

1. Mix the soy and oyster sauces, the mirin, chilli, garlic and cornflour in a medium bowl.

2. Add the chicken and leave to marinate in the fridge for at least 20 minutes and up to 8 hours.

3. Heat the oil in a non-stick wok over a high heat until smoking slightly (if using 1-cal cooking spray, the temperature should be a little lower).

4. Stir-fry all the vegetables (including the ginger, but not the lettuce) for 2 minutes.

5. Add the chicken and the marinade and stir-fry for a further 3–4 minutes, until the chicken is cooked through and the sauce is thickened. If necessary add 2–3 tablespoons of water to keep the sauce thick but not burned. Season to taste with salt and pepper.

6. Put a tablespoon of the chicken mixture in the centre of each lettuce leaf and garnish with a little coriander. Wrap up into a roll and eat with your fingers!

Kate says: I love how Fiona has adapted one of her favourites and made it into the healthiest possible takeaway. All that chopping burns a few extra calories on Fast Day, too! I love these with tofu – just marinate it in the same way as the chicken, but leave out the oyster sauce if you're a vegetarian.

SWEET POTATO FALAFEL POCKETS

Falafels are such great street food – my favourites used to be the ones freshly fried in a stall next to Shepherds Bush Market in London. Then I discovered these: all the crunch and spicy flavours of falafel, without the calorie disaster that is deep-frying. The ras al hanout spice mix, which includes ginger, paprika, allspice, cardamom, mace and even rose petals, adds a warming, Middle-Eastern hit.

You can make a batch of the falafel and they will keep cooked in the fridge for up to four days. They also freeze well; once cooked, pack them into freezer-proof boxes and freeze for up to a month. Defrost and warm in the microwave (or oven) until piping hot and then serve as below.

Serves 6
Calories per falafel: 44
Calories per serving (4 falafel): 334 with pitta; 197 without
Preparation time: 25 minutes, plus chilling
Cooking time: 35 minutes

3 sweet potatoes (about 750g) *675 cals*
1 tsp ras al hanout *5 cals*
2 cloves garlic, finely chopped *8 cals*
2 tsp ground cumin *10 cals*
3 tbsp chopped fresh coriander leaves *15 cals*
squeeze lemon juice
100g plain white or gram (chickpea) flour, plus extra if needed *335 cals*

1-cal cooking spray
6 wholemeal pitta breads or flatbreads *580 cals*
6 tbsp reduced-fat hummus *77 cals* (or try the Roasted Squash Hummus on page 240)
2 Little Gem lettuces, shredded *20–30 cals*
salt and pepper

1. Place the sweet potatoes in the microwave and cook on High for 8–10 minutes, until tender (or cook them in a preheated oven at 180°C/350°F/Gas mark 4 for 45 minutes, until soft). Leave to cool a little, then peel.

2. Put the potato, ras al hanout, garlic, cumin, chopped coriander, a little squeeze of lemon juice and the flour in a large bowl. Go easy on the lemon juice, as you don't want the mix too wet or it will be difficult to roll into balls. Season with salt and pepper, then mash until smooth.

3. Using a tablespoon and lightly oiled hands, shape the mixture into about 24 balls. If the mixture is too wet add a little more flour. Chill for 20 minutes or until firm to the touch.

4. Preheat the grill to medium-high. Arrange the falafel on a lightly greased baking sheet. Grill for 10 minutes until the base of the falafels are golden brown, then flip over and bake for 10 minutes more, until golden brown all over.

5. To serve, warm the pitta breads or flatbreads, split them open horizontally, spread each with a tablespoon of hummus, scatter with a little lettuce and top with four hot falafel balls.

VIETNAMESE PRAWN SUMMER ROLLS

I made these in Vietnam five years ago, at a cookery school in the beautiful town of Hoi Ann, where I also had a red silk dress made (I later got mugged in the dress in Ho Chi Minh City, but that's another story). But as the weight crept on, I could no longer wear the only dress I've ever had made to measure. First the zip wouldn't do up without effort. Then the seams were under serious pressure. Now the dress fits again. Actually, it's a little loose. And the summer rolls are every bit as fresh-tasting as I remember them (you can use a little fried tofu or some extra veg like carrot or courgette in place of the prawns for a completely veggie version).

Makes 8
Calories per roll with sauce: 84
Preparation time: 25 minutes

50g cooked fine rice noodles *97 cals*

5cm piece cucumber, cut into matchsticks *5 cals*

1 Little Gem lettuce, finely shredded *15 cals*

2 tbsp chopped fresh mint leaves *10 cals*

2 tbsp chopped fresh coriander leaves *10 cals*

2 tbsp chopped fresh Thai or normal basil leaves *10 cals*

1 tbsp toasted sesame seeds *96 cals*

8 x large round rice paper wrappers (available from large supermarkets or Asian stores) *160 cals*

16 large cooked peeled prawns, halved lengthways *140 cals*

For the dipping sauce

1 tbsp soy sauce *6 cals*
juice of ½ lime *10 cals*
2 tsp toasted sesame oil *90 cals*
1 tsp fish sauce *3 cals*
1 tsp soft brown sugar *15 cals*
½ red chilli, deseeded and finely chopped *2–6 cals*

1. Place the cooked noodles in a large bowl and chop roughly. Add the cucumber sticks, shredded lettuce, mint, coriander, basil and toasted sesame seeds and mix together.

2. Whisk together all the ingredients for the dipping sauce in a bowl. Add 1–2 tablespoons of the sauce to the noodle mix and stir together. Pour the rest of the dipping sauce into a small bowl and set aside.

3. Dip a rice paper wrapper in a bowl of hot water for 10 seconds, until soft and pliable. Place on a damp board and then put 4 prawn halves in a line across the middle. Top with a tablespoon of the noodle mixture. Fold over the sides to secure the filling and then roll up tightly into a spring-roll shape. Repeat until you have used up all the filling and rice papers. Chill until ready to serve.

4. Serve the rolls with the dipping sauce on the side.

TUNA NIÇOISE WRAPS

The classic Mediterranean salad in a wrap. These are *so* satisfying and I swear they taste of sunshine: they are extra-good warm if you're serving them fresh.

Serves 2
Calories per serving: 298
Preparation time: 15 minutes
Cooking time: 10 minutes

1 egg *78 cals*
50g green beans, trimmed *14 cals*
2 tbsp light mayonnaise *24 cals*
2 wholemeal tortilla wraps, warmed *218 cals*
30g baby spinach leaves *8 cals*
1 x 185g tin tuna in spring water, drained *183 cals*
1 tbsp small capers, drained *5 cals*
1 large ripe tomato, cut into 8 pieces *20 cals*
20g drained and rinsed pitted black olives, halved *45 cals*
salt and pepper

1. Place the egg in a small saucepan of boiling water, bring back to the boil and then boil for 8 minutes. Cool quickly in cold water, peel and then cut into 8 wedges.

2. Meanwhile, blanch the beans in boiling water for 2–3 minutes. Drain, refresh/dip in cold water to stop them cooking further and set aside.

3. Spread half a tablespoon of mayonnaise over each tortilla wrap and divide the spinach leaves between them.

4. Mix the other tablespoon of mayonnaise with the tuna and capers and season well with salt and pepper.

5. Divide the tuna mix between the wraps and then top with the sliced egg, sliced tomato, olives and beans. Fold up the bottom edge of the wrap (to seal in the filling) and then roll up tightly. Wrap in foil if you are not eating it straight away and keep chilled until ready to eat.

AVOCADO WRAPS OR LITTLE GEM 'OPEN SANDWICHES'

In my own personal sandwich Top of the Pops (something I've spent a long time debating), the Pret a Manger Avocado and Herb Salad Wrap is a serious contender. However, at 460+ calories per wrap, it's not good for Fast Day lunching, so I thought I'd invent my own.

Avocados are highly nutritious (see page 172) but also quite high in calories, so this recipe uses half an avocado – or you could also try the smaller 'baby' avocados. The unused half can go brown after cutting; keep the stone in, and squeezing over some lemon juice before wrapping in cling film will reduce that.

You can also cut back on the cals by using lettuce leaves as the 'wrap' – or split the filling between two tortilla wraps, with extra salad, for a perfect takeaway lunch for two (works out at 212 cals per tortills wrap).

Serves 1 (makes 1 tortilla wrap or several lettuce cups or wraps)
Calories per serving: 324 in tortilla wrap; 229 in lettuce cup/
    wrap
Preparation time: 10 minutes

½ small Hass avocado *110–140 cals*
squeeze lemon juice *3 cals*
1 tortilla wrap (*100–200 cals*) OR
larger leaves from romaine or iceberg lettuce or smaller Little
    Gem lettuce leaves *5 cals or 10–15 cals*
3–4cm piece cucumber, thinly sliced *10 cals*

small handful mixed fresh basil, parsley and rocket leaves *5 cals*

3 cherry tomatoes, quartered *9 cals*

10g Parmesan cheese shavings (use a potato peeler, then
    crumble into more pieces) *42 cals*

5g pine nuts, dry-fried *35 cals*

2 tsp Creamy Herb Dressing (see page 315) *10 cals*

salt and pepper

1. Remove the avocado peel and stone and slice the avocado into thin slices.
   Squeeze over a little lemon juice.

2. Open up the wrap or lay the lettuce leaves on a board. Layer the avocado
   and other ingredients along the centre or bottom half of the wrap or
   lettuce leaves. Drizzle the dressing between layers of ingredients.

3. Fold up the bottom edge of the wrap (to seal in the filling) and then roll
   up tightly. Cut in half, to serve. If using lettuce leaves, carefully wrap
   up and secure with a cocktail stick. If using Little Gem leaves, you could
   leave them unwrapped and serve as 'open sandwiches'! They taste best
   fresh, but you can refrigerate them till you're ready to eat.

GRANOLA SQUARES

These tempting squares are packed with good things and the sweetness of the fruit is perfectly balanced by the nuts and oats. I wouldn't recommend making these *every* Fast Day and you do have to be very strong-willed not to scoff the lot, but they keep for a week in a well-sealed tin. They would be great if it's your turn to take some goodies to work and they're a lot better for you than a chocolate chip cookie!

NB: Reduced-fat butter allows you to keep the taste and moistness of butter with a lower calorie count. Do check the labels as calorie counts vary.

Makes 16 squares
Calories per square: 148
Preparation time: 15 minutes
Cooking time: 25 minutes

150g reduced-fat butter, plus extra for greasing *566–855 cals*
150g pitted Medjool dates, chopped *430 cals*
3 tbsp apple juice *19 cals*
30g toasted whole almonds or hazelnuts, finely chopped *183 or 200 cals*
50g sultanas or dried cherries *150 cals*
50g dried apricots, finely chopped *125 cals*
225g rolled oats *799 cals*
15g desiccated coconut *95 cals*

1. Preheat the oven to 190°C/375°F/Gas mark 5. Lightly grease and line a shallow 20cm-square tin with non-stick baking paper.

2. Put the dates and apple juice in a food processor and whizz until smooth.

3. Melt the butter in a large non-stick saucepan over a low heat. Add the date purée and all the other ingredients. Stir well, then press into the prepared tin and level the surface. Bake for 20–25 minutes, until just golden on top.

4. Remove from the oven and cool for 10 minutes. Cut into 16 squares in the tin. Cool completely before turning out and cutting through again to separate.

BERRY BLAST SMOOTHIE

Shop-bought smoothies tend to be tricky, as you don't know what's gone into them and you can't control the blood sugar rebound that can make you hungry after eating fruit.

Making your own allows you to control the ingredients. Using almond milk in place of skimmed cow's milk will reduce the insulin release that we're trying to avoid. If you can 'spare' the calories, then either a 5g portion of sesame seeds (*32 cals*) or ground almonds (*31 cals*) added after blending will make this an even more satisfying meal in a glass.

Serves 1
Calories per serving: 161 with skimmed milk; 139 with
    almond milk
Preparation time: 5 minutes

    1 small banana *89 cals*
    50g frozen or fresh berries *19 cals*
    ½ tsp Manuka or clear honey *10 cals*
    1 tbsp vanilla yoghurt *8–15 cals*
    100ml skimmed or almond milk *35 or 13 cals*

1. Place all the ingredients in a blender, adding a few ice cubes if you are using fresh fruit, and blend until smooth. Pass through a sieve into a tall glass, and drink straight away with a straw.

STICKY BANANA AND DATE BREAD

I adore Medjool dates; they're as sweet as toffee and work so well with the bananas in this easy-to-make tea bread. Sundays are baking days at home and I love to make something we can enjoy all week: when I make this, the house smells almost like bananas and custard, thanks to the vanilla flavours. A slice of this loaf makes a great high-energy treat to take to work on a Fast Day. Just make sure you only take one piece! It will keep for up to four days in a well-sealed container.

Makes 12 slices
Calories per slice: 185
Preparation time: 15 minutes
Cooking time: 50 minutes–1 hour

85g reduced-fat butter, plus extra to grease *320–485 cals*
125g light muscovado or soft brown sugar *480 cals*
1 egg, beaten *78 cals*
1 tsp vanilla extract *12 cals*
4 small very ripe bananas, peeled (peeled weight about 350g)
   356 cals
75g Medjool pitted dates, chopped *215 cals*
225g self-raising white flour *753 cals*
1 tsp baking powder *5 cals*

1. Preheat the oven to 180°C/350°F/Gas mark 4. Beat the butter and sugar together using an electric hand whisk until pale and fluffy. Then beat in the egg and vanilla extract.

2. Mash the bananas in a large bowl using a potato masher, and then stir into the sugar mixture along with the chopped dates.

3. Sift the flour and baking powder over the banana mixture and fold together gently.

4. Lightly grease and line a 900g-loaf tin with non-stick baking paper. Spoon the banana mixture into the prepared tin and level the surface.

5. Bake for 50–60 minutes until golden brown on top and a skewer inserted into the centre comes out clean.

6. Remove from the oven and leave the bread to cool in the tin for 10–15 minutes before turning out and cooling on a wire rack. Slice carefully so you get 12 slices out of the loaf – or your calories per portion will rise!

THE 5:2 LUNCHBOX

There are lots of great ideas in this book for dishes that can work for work! Take soups, stews and curries in air-tight plastic boxes and reheat in the microwave. It's much cheaper than buying ready meals or eating from the canteen.

Cool lunches

- Banana Oat Muffins (see pages 48–49), Vanilla Granola Pots with Berry Compote (see pages 50–51), Mushroom and Spinach Omelette Muffins (see pages 52–53) are all easily transported.

- Most of the Salads from Salad Days (see pages 164–201) will work well to go. Keep the dressing in a separate pot and dress at work to avoid soggy salad leaves.

Hot dinners

- All the recipes from Super Soups (see pages 168–99) can be taken to work in a microwaveable pot to be reheated.

- Thai curry (see pages 108–109), Lizzie's Harira (see pages 106–107), Kate's Saag Paneer (see page 113), Skinny Chilli con Carne (see pages 125–126), Beef and Ale Stew (see pages 142–143), Best Vegetarian Cottage Pie (see pages 153–154) can all be reheated in a microwave at work.

Lunchbox Legends

Even the lowest-calorie bought sandwiches can knock a big hole in your 5:2 calorie limit — not to mention your budget. So, taking a sandwich or wrap to work will save you money *and* cut the pounds.

Wraps/breads

- **Wraps or tortillas:** corn or wheat wraps can save on calories when compared with two slices of normal bread. They also come in packs that keep for several months so are a good standby. They range from 100 calories to about 200, so make sure you check the label.

- **Warburton's Thins:** these are a recent discovery for me but they're like mini-panini breads, which split down the middle and are 100 calories total. They are surprisingly nice, and good for toasted sandwiches, too.

- **Lettuce leaves:** see the recipes for Fiona's Asian Chicken Lettuce Wraps, and Avocado Little Gem 'Open Sandwiches' (pages 211–212 and 220–221) for more information, but large and crunchy leaves that form a kind of pocket or bowl can work well when the filling is the star.

Famously Good Fillings

All of these fillings are delicious and work well with the wraps and breads listed above. Use the Calorie Counter (see pages 338–347) to calculate the portion size that keeps you under your Fast Day limit.

- Roasted Squash Hummus (see page 240) with half a sliced red pepper *94 cals*

- Baba Ganoush (see page 74) with 15g rocket leaves *242 cals*

- 1 slice reduced-fat mature cheese (*60–75 cals*) OR 30g/2 tablespoons any flavour low-fat cream cheese (*44 cals*), with 1 sliced cooked beetroot (either in vinegar or water, 50g/*22 cals*) with a few watercress leaves

- Half a 130g tin of tuna in spring water (*64 cals*), mixed with 1 chopped spring onion (*2 cals*) and Yoghurt Dressing (see pages 117–118)

- 50g sliced cooked chicken (*83 cals*) with a tablespoon of Sweet and Sour Balsamic Dressing (see page 315), a few thin slices of red onion (*5 cals*) and 3 halved cherry tomatoes (*9–12 cals*)

- 20g low-fat feta cheese (*36 cals*) with ½ sliced tomato (*8 cals*), 5 drained and pitted black olives (*25 cals*), a few red onion slices (*5 cals*), ½ a green pepper (*15 cals*), sliced, and any dressing (see pages 314–317).

- 1 sliced hard-boiled egg (*78 cals*) with ½ a sliced cucumber (*15 cals*).

5:2 Know-How

FASTING ON A BUDGET

One of the best things about 5:2 is that it saves you money. Not only are you eating less and therefore spending less on food, but also you don't need to buy any of the supplements, shakes or other specialist foods that some diets demand. However, if your budget is tight, then there are ways to make your Fast Days cheaper than chips, and also a lot healthier!

- **Making food from scratch** is the biggest step you can take to cut costs. My Tomato and Lentil Soup (see pages 87–88) costs around 85p for two very generous portions – a shop-bought 'fresh' soup with similar ingredients will be roughly £1.99.

- **Batch cooking.** Making more than you need and then freezing individual portions for later means you're less likely to succumb to ready-meals, and you can also cut down on your energy bills if you reheat in the microwave.

- **Choosing seasonal ingredients** that are grown in the UK or Europe tends to be cheaper, and have less of an environmental impact, than buying food flown thousands of miles. Seasonal fruit and veg also tend to be tastier (if you've ever tasted an April strawberry that's more green/yellow than red, you'll know what I mean). Try finding a local greengrocer or market stall where you can ask what's in seaon or research veg box deliveries in your area (see pages 202–205).

- **New stores, lower prices.** Try shopping around for good bargains. Shops specialising in ethnic foods will often have the lowest prices for spices, vegtables or staples like lentils or couscous.

- **Frozen and tinned food** is often better value, and can be at least as good nutritionally as fresh because it's been preserved at the point of picking, rather than having to travel to shops in refrigerated lorries. Peas, sweetcorn and spinach are great examples of low-cost and high convenience foods.

- **Using leftovers is thrifty and satisfying.** I've been making my own stock since starting 5:2, and I really like saving veg scraps that are past their best for this purpose (see pages 316–318). Stir-fries, grilled veg and soups are also good for using up produce. Sell-by dates are advisory, so if a food a day or two past the date looks and smells OK, it should be safe to cook. However, take Use-By dates seriously; they're there to protect your health.

- **Cheaper cuts of meat** make fabulous stews and casseroles, often with much more flavour than the expensive cuts. And they add so much depth to stock, too.

- **Buy less.** After starting 5:2, I found it hard to get used to how much less food – especially convenience food – I was using and my freezer was soon at bursting point. Review your regular shopping list to reflect your healthier habits!

CHAPTER SEVEN

5:2 On Tour

A TASTE OF HOLIDAYS AROUND THE GLOBE

I wonder what percentage of diets are inspired by holidays – either by planning for your beach body, or by facing the reality of the holiday snaps when you get home.

The photo of me looking my biggest pre-5:2 shows me trying to hide behind a flowery sarong (you can see it on my website). It's the shameful expression on my face that jumps out at me now. I felt worse than I looked, and it's a reminder for me of how much better I now feel about my body and about enjoying food.

Whatever stage you're at in your healthy eating journey, this chapter is all about capturing those holiday flavours. We've a taste of the Mediterranean with pasta and risotto dishes, Greek mezze and even pizza; a little Thai spice with prawns skewers; a stroganoff rich in Eastern paprika; and a Mexican twist that makes our veggie bean burgers hot stuff. *Bon voyage, amigos*!

RECICES

BECCA'S PERFECT PIZZA

GREEK MEZZE OF ROASTED SQUASH HUMMUS, TZATZIKI
AND BABA GANOUSH

BOTTOM-OF-THE-FRIDGE FRITTATA

MUSHROOM STROGANOFF

GARAM MASALA SPICED MUSHROOMS

CHICKEN, LEMON AND OLIVE TAGINE

GREEK SPRING LAMB STEW

THAI PRAWN SKEWERS WITH GRIDDLED COURGETTE,
PEA AND MINT SALAD

LEMON AND ASPARAGUS RISOTTO

CORIANDER, LIME AND CHILLI PRAWN PASTA

HOT SMOKED SALMON AND WATERCRESS LINGUINI

SPICY MEXICAN BEAN BURGERS

5:2 Lives

BECCA'S MARATHON JOURNEY

'I'm beginning to feel more confident about myself and the skin I'm in.'

As Becca Blake from Gloucester celebrated the New Year, she knew this was going to be the big one. It was the year she was turning 30, and the year she planned to tackle both the Great North Run and the Yorkshire marathon. Yet she didn't feel in the best shape to tackle it.

'I was unhappy with my body. Clothes were starting to feel tight and I was aware of my BMI and body fat percentage creeping up. I want to be fit at 30 in every sense.'

Care assistant Becca, who lives with her partner, had struggled with restricted diets. 'I wasn't a fan of being told what I could and couldn't eat, and so much thought went into planning the weeks ahead. I'd heard about 5:2 and looked for a book on my Kindle. I found Kate's, downloaded it, read it in a day and haven't looked back since.'

As a care assistant, Becca works long days in a physically demanding job – and is also training for her runs. But it's proving easy to stick to 5:2. 'I work long shifts, from 8 a.m to 8 p.m. and I normally fast on a workday because it's so busy. It fits in easily with work, but I'm always listening to my body and if I feel it's not the right day for a fast I can easily come off it.'

When it comes to the running, 'I often train on an empty stomach in the mornings anyway, so on a Fast Day it works fine for me and before work fits in nicely. When the distance increases, then I will start doing longer runs on Feast Days and only after I've had a good breakfast of porridge (which is what I'd do on a race day).'

It's her shrinking measurements that have made the biggest difference to Becca. In under eight weeks, she'd lost 9cm (3.5 in) from her waist, 7.5cm (3 in) from her hips, 5.5cm (2.25 in) from her chest and 5cm (2 in) from each thigh. Not to mention 5kg (11 lb) towards her 12.75kg (28 lb) target.

'I can now fit comfortably into a pair of trousers I haven't worn for six years – that includes zipping them up and sitting down in them! Plus my mood is better; I find that I feel less stressed when I'm at work and I'm beginning to feel more confident about myself and the skin I'm in.'

Becca's Fast Day Diary

Breakfast is at 7 a.m. and is a cup of tea with milk (I can't go without tea and don't like black tea). Lunch, at 2 p.m. is homemade root veg soup (I use a pack of root veg from the supermarket), a Weight Watcher's meal or a low-calorie meal from home. I eat dinner at 6 p.m. and it's usually a Quorn sausage with sweet potato and salad, or my pizza (see pages 238–239) with whichever topping I fancy that day.

I finish with a Ski mousse. I keep hydrated with water and two or three cups of tea.

Feast Day Secrets

I don't count calories on Feast Days and allow myself some treats; if I fancy something then I have it. I have noticed my appetite has reduced; I don't snack as much and often leave food on my plate (our dogs are very pleased about that!). I tend to have a lot of stews during the winter, and in the summer, I'll be tucking into fresh salads. My sweet tooth has always been my problem but now I don't feel guilty or deny myself and I eat much less. I usually have porridge with mixed berries for breakfast, eggs on toast for lunch and a stew or casserole with veg for dinner (and the odd takeaway, too).

Favourite Foods

Anything I bake. Cupcakes, Victoria sponge, gingerbread or scones are a big favourite (they hide in the tin on Fast Days though). I love Chinese food, and can still have the odd takeaway and not feel guilty at all.

Fast Day Top Tips

- Do not enter the supermarket on a Fast Day; it's full of temptations.

- If you feel awful on a Fast Day and like you really cannot do it, don't worry about it and just try it the next day. I originally stuck with rigid Fast Days but I have become much more flexible about it so it can fit in with long shifts,

and will be moving them around to fit in with longer
training sessions.

The Best Thing About 5:2

I don't feel at all guilty for eating any 'naughty' food like
biscuits or chocolate. If I feel like I want something on a Fast
Day I just tell myself that I can have plenty of it the next day,
and by the next day I've usually forgotten about it. In myself I
feel great and full of energy.

BECCA'S PERFECT PIZZA

Becca says: 'The beauty of this dish is that it's just like a small pizza and the toppings can be adapted to suit your mood. Also, my partner can have his pizza with all the calories and I can have my pizza with fewer calories, which means our meals are the same and we're still eating together. I feel less like I'm missing out than if I had a salad and he had a pizza. I play around with toppings like sweetcorn, sliced mushrooms and my most recent find: sliced tinned ham, which is low in calories.'

Serves 1
Calories per serving: 246
Preparation time: 5 minutes
Cooking time: 15 minutes

50g half-fat mozzarella cheese *85–95 cals*
25g low-fat feta cheese *45 cals*
20g tomato purée *6–23 cals*
1 small white flour tortilla wrap *90–115 cals (depending on brand)*
5 cherry tomatoes, halved *12 cals*
30g baby spinach leaves *8 cals*
pepper
fresh basil leaves, to serve

1. Preheat the oven to 200°C/400°F/Gas mark 6. Preheat a baking sheet in the oven for 5 minutes.

2. Slice or tear the mozzarella into pieces and crumble the feta with your fingers.

3. Spread the tomato purée evenly across the tortilla base, leaving a 1cm (½ in) border around the edge. Scatter over the cheeses and tomato halves evenly. Season with pepper.

4. Place on the preheated baking sheet and bake in the oven for 10 minutes, until the cheeses have melted and the base is crisp, but not burned.

5. Either remove from the oven, scatter the spinach over the top and return to the oven for 3–4 minutes to wilt the leaves, *or* serve with the spinach on the side as a salad. You can dress the salad with balsamic vinegar (around 10 calories per tablespoon) or one of the low-fat dressings from pages 312–315.

6. Garnish with torn fresh basil leaves just before serving.

Kate says: Becca's pizza makes me very happy – especially when it comes to varying the toppings. My version is based on my favourite 'Holy Cheeses' Feast Day Pizza from my local delivery company with low-fat feta, some dollops of Light Philadelphia, the thinnest slivers of Cheddar or Parmesan, plus plenty of sliced red onion. Yum. I need one right now!

GREEK MEZZE OF ROASTED SQUASH HUMMUS, TZATZIKI AND BABA GANOUSH

I love dips and these are three of my favourites. They look wonderful served together (no wonder they're our cover stars!).

Regular hummus is surprisingly high in calories and fat, but adding squash makes it go further. There are a couple of interesting ingredients used in the dips: baharat is used in Arabian, Turkish and Iranian cooking and contains nine different spices including paprika, coriander, cinnamon and cloves. Pomegranate molasses adds a wonderful sweetness to the smoky aubergine in the Baba Ganoush. Both will be cheapest from Middle-Eastern shops.

Serve the dips at room temperature with your choice of toasted wholemeal pitta bread or crispbreads, baby carrots, radishes, chopped peppers, cucumber sticks or sugar snap peas. All the dips serve four.

Roasted Squash Hummus
Calories per serving: 94
Preparation time: 20 minutes
Cooking time: 30 minutes

- 1 small butternut squash (about 400g), peeled, deseeded and chopped *160 cals*
- 1-cal cooking spray
- 2 cloves garlic, unpeeled and bashed *8 cals*
- 3cm piece fresh root ginger, peeled and grated *3 cals*
- ½ tsp hot paprika, plus extra to serve *2 cals*

2 tsp baharat, or 1 tsp ground cumin and 1 tsp ground
    coriander *10–15 cals*
2 tsp light tahini *60 cals*
200g tinned chickpeas, drained and rinsed *130 cals*
zest of ½ lemon plus 2 tbsp lemon juice *4 cals*
salt and pepper

1. Preheat the oven to 200°C/400°F/Gas mark 6. Place the squash in a
   large bowl, spray with a little 1-cal cooking spray and add the garlic and
   ginger. Sprinkle over the spices and season well with salt and pepper.

2. Tip into a large baking tray and roast, turning occasionally, for 30
   minutes, or until tender and turning golden. Set aside for a couple of
   minutes to cool.

3. Tip the squash into a blender. Squeeze the garlic from its skin and add to
   the squash (discard the skin). Add the tahini, chickpeas and lemon juice
   and zest. Blend with 2 tablespoons of water until coarsely blended.

4. Spoon into a serving dish and sprinkle with a little paprika before serving.

Tzatziki
Calories per serving: 36
Preparation time: 10 minutes

10cm piece cucumber, peeled, deseeded and cut into small
    cubes *20 cals*
200g fat-free natural yoghurt *110 cals*
2 tbsp chopped fresh mint, plus mint sprigs to garnish *10 cals*
¼ tsp ground cumin *2 cals*
½ small clove garlic, crushed *2 cals*

squeeze lime juice
salt and pepper

1. Mix together all the ingredients and season well with salt and pepper. Spoon into a serving dish and garnish with mint sprigs.

Baba Ganoush

Calories per serving: 74
Preparation time: 10 minutes
Cooking time: 20 minutes

2 large aubergines 36 cals
1 clove garlic, crushed *4 cals*
juice 1 small lemon *8 cals*
1 tbsp light tahini 90 cals
1 tbsp light olive oil *135 cals*
10g pomegranate seeds *8 cals*
1 tsp pomegranate molasses *15 cals*

1. Preheat the grill to high. Prick the aubergines all over with a fork then grill for 15–20 minutes, turning occasionally, until the aubergines are black all over and tender.

2. Leave to cool slightly, then remove and discard the black skin. Scoop the aubergine flesh into a large bowl and roughly mash with a fork.

3. Add the garlic, lemon juice, tahini, oil and a splash of water, and mix together until it forms a rough paste.

4. Scatter with pomegranate seeds and drizzle with pomegranate molasses.

BOTTOM-OF-THE-FRIDGE FRITTATA

A frittata is like an Italian grilled or baked omelette. Grilling helps the topping caramelise, which adds extra flavour. Frittatas are perfect for lunchboxes, and they are a great way of using up tired bits of veg or unused beans or cooked meats lurking in your fridge. As a rule, I'd aim for one or two types of vegetable, a herb or spice, plus one protein e.g. cheese, sausages or fish. Anymore and the flavours may be muddled. A generous amount of seasoning stops the eggs tasting bland.

It's actually a little easier to make a double quantity, as the mix will fill a small frying pan, so save time and double up the recipe. Make half for brunch and half for later, but bear in mind that it will take a little longer to cook. The recipe is similar to the Omelette breakfast muffins in Chapter 1 and you bake them individually the same way.

Serves 1
Calories per serving: 217 (but will vary according to what's in the bottom of your fridge!)
Preparation time: 5 minutes
Cooking time: 15 minutes

  1 cal-spray
  75–100g mixed veg, e.g. mushrooms, spring onions, onions, green beans, peppers, spinach and fresh herbs including fresh thyme, mint and parsley *approx. 20–30 cals depending on what you choose*
  2 eggs *156 cals*

small handful fresh herbs, chopped *5 cals*

20g low-fat feta cheese *36 cals*

salt and pepper

Optional extras

20g chopped tinned ham *17–23 cals*

20g smoked salmon *44 cals*

30g tinned cannellini beans, drained and rinsed *25 cals*

½ leftover cooked Quorn sausage *35 cals*

2 cooked cocktail sausages *40 cals*

chilli flakes

1 tsp green pesto *23 cals*

1. Chop all the veg into small, even chunks or slices.

2. Spray a small non-stick frying pan with 1-cal cooking spray. Fry the veg and any non-cheese 'extras' over a medium heat for about 3–5 minutes to soften and caramelise slightly. Remove from the pan and allow to cool. Drain off any excess liquid once cooled; vegetables like courgettes will 'leak', which may affect the flavour and consistency of your finished frittata.

3. Break the eggs into a bowl and beat lightly with a fork. Season well with salt and pepper. Add in any additional herbs or seasonings, plus the cooked veg mix.

4. Preheat the grill to high. Pour the egg mixture into a grill-proof frying pan and use a spatula to distribute the veg evenly. Cook over a low heat for 2–3 minutes, until the bottom is brown.

5. Scatter over the feta (as you're not using much, it's nice to have that on the top) and cook under the grill for 3–4 minutes, until the top is set.

(If your pan isn't grill-proof, when the bottom is set, place a slightly larger plate on top of the pan and carefully turn the pan over. Slide the frittata back into the pan, uncooked-side down. Don't worry if it breaks as you turn it, it'll set again. It'll take another 3–4 minutes to cook through.)

For mini frittatas

1. Preheat the oven to 180°C/350°/Gas mark 4. Spray two holes of a muffin tin with a little 1-cal cooking spray. I find a deep silicon mould works best for these as the muffins are easier to remove and also the mix doesn't bubble up over the tin.

2. Mix the cheese into the egg and vegetable mix (as before) and divide the mix between the muffin holes.

3. Bake for 14–16 minutes, until the tops are browned. Remove while warm to reduce the chance of sticking.

Suggestions: This frittata is great served with a green salad or my Smoky and Peppery Salsa (see pages 310–311).

To serve later, allow the frittata to cool, then store in an airtight container in the fridge. Reheat in the microwave for 30–40 seconds on High.

This also makes a tasty sandwich filling, sliced and used to fill a crusty roll on a Feast Day.

MUSHROOM STROGANOFF

Mushrooms, garlic and crème fraîche – no wonder this is one of my favourites! It really doesn't taste like it is this low in calories. You can make double quantities and chill one portion without the crème fraîche. It will keep for up to two days in the fridge. If you prefer your mushrooms with a kick, try the spicy version on page 248!

Serves 1
Calories per serving: 70
Preparation time: 5 minutes
Cooking time: 15 minutes

2g dried porcini mushrooms *5 cals*
50ml boiling water
1-cal cooking spray
½ onion, peeled and finely chopped *19 cals*
1 clove garlic, chopped or crushed *4 cals*
½ teaspoon paprika (or try smoked paprika) *3 cals*
100g mushrooms, chopped or sliced (use your favourite variety, but chestnut mushrooms work well in this dish) *13 cals*
squeeze lemon juice
1 tbsp reduced-fat crème fraîche *26 cals*
salt and pepper
fresh parsley leaves or chives, to garnish

1. Soak the porcini mushrooms in the boiling water for at least 10 minutes while you cook the other vegetables.

2. Spray a small non-stick pan with 1-cal cooking spray. Cook the onion for 2–3 minutes, until softened. Add the garlic and paprika and cook for another minute.

3. Add the chopped fresh mushrooms and a squeeze of lemon juice (this will add flavour and also helps prevent the mushrooms from sticking to the pan until they begin to release their juices). Cook over a medium heat for 5 minutes.

4. Chop or tear the soaked mushrooms into smaller pieces. Add these and the soaking liquid to the pan and heat for 4–5 minutes, until the sauce starts to thicken. Stir in 4 tablespoons of water, if necessary, to help loosen the sauce.

5. Remove from the heat. If serving immediately, stir in the crème fraîche and season with salt and pepper. Serve topped with chopped parsley or chives. Perfect with Cauliflower Rice or Courgette Pasta (see pages 303–304 or 321–322).

Variations: Use as a stuffing for sweet peppers. Cut 1 red or yellow pepper in half (15 cals), remove the core and seeds and grill, cut-side down, for 5 minutes. Add the mushroom mix (without the crème fraîche) and grill for 2 minutes. Top with crème fraîche just before serving. These are great with a crisp green salad.

GARAM MASALA SPICED MUSHROOMS

This variation on the stroganoff recipe uses a warming garam masala spice blend.

Serves 1
Calories per serving: 71
Preparation time: 5 minutes
Cooking time: 15 minutes

   1-cal cooking spray
   4–5 small spring onions, chopped into small pieces *6 cals*
   100g mixed mushrooms, chopped roughly (a few shiitake
      would work well as part of the mix) *13 cals*
   ¼ tsp each of ginger, turmeric and ground coriander OR, for a
      sweeter flavour, ¼ tsp garam masala (*5 cals*)
   pinch chilli flakes
   squeeze lemon juice *3 cals*
   200g tin chopped tomatoes *36 cals*
   salt and pepper
   1 tbsp fat-free Greek yoghurt, to serve 8 cals
   fresh coriander leaves, to garnish

1. Spray a small non-stick saucepan with 2 sprays of 1-cal cooking spray. Cook the spring onions over a medium heat for 2–3 minutes – it doesn't matter if they brown a little.

2. Add the mushrooms, spices, chilli and lemon juice and fry for 2 minutes.

3. Add the tomatoes and turn up the heat so that the mix begins to bubble. Cook for about 10 minutes, until the sauce starts to thicken, stirring

occasionally to make sure it doesn't stick. Add a splash of water if necessary at any point to loosen.

4. Serve with the yoghurt and garnish with the coriander.

Variation: Add 75g cubed firm tofu (*64–134 cals*) at the same stage as the mushrooms for a more substantial dish. Garam masala is often used towards the end of cooking to add warmth, but it won't do any harm to add it earlier as we do here.

CHICKEN, LEMON AND OLIVE TAGINE

You don't need a Moroccan tagine pot to produce the most tender and fragrant chicken this side of Marrakech. The preserved lemons, saffron and olives make this a very special dish that gives you so much taste for your calories. Try to allow some extra calories for couscous to soak up the flavours.

Serves 4
Calories per serving: 406 with couscous; 312 without
Preparation time: 30 minutes
Cooking time: 1 hour 10 minutes

1-cal cooking spray
1 red onion, peeled and sliced *38 cals*
2 cloves garlic, finely chopped *8 cals*
1 tsp ground cumin *5 cals*
1 tsp ground coriander *5 cals*
2 tsp ground ginger *10 cals*
1 cinnamon stick
8 chicken thighs, skin removed, seasoned with salt and pepper *880 cals*
500ml hot chicken stock *20 cals*
pinch saffron
200g large green pitted olives *213 cals*
2 small preserved lemons, flesh removed and peel finely shredded *10 cals*
200g baby spinach leaves *50 cals*
2 tbsp chopped fresh flat-leaf parsley *10 cals*

salt and pepper
100g cooked couscous, to serve (optional) *376 cals*

1. Spray a large heavy-bottomed casserole with 1-cal cooking spray. Add the onion and a splash of water, season with salt and pepper and cook over a medium heat for 5 minutes, until softened. Add the garlic and spices and fry for another 2 minutes.

2. Add the cinnamon stick, chicken, hot stock and saffron. Stir well and bring to the boil, then turn down the heat, cover and simmer for 45 minutes. Top up with a little water if necessary; don't let the pan go dry.

3. Add the olives and preserved lemon and cook for 10–15 minutes. Remove the cinnamon stick before stirring through the baby spinach. Scatter the dish with parsley and serve hot with couscous or some lightly steamed green vegetables.

GREEK SPRING LAMB STEW

This dish makes me think of families eating lunch on tables spilling out of a taverna in the spring sunshine, but even if the weather's not good enough for eating *al fresco*, this is still a great, low-calorie family meal. The secret is in the long, slow cooking, so that the lamb and vegetables melt in the mouth!

Serves 4
Calories per serving: 239 (don't forget to add calories for any rice, couscous or green vegtables to serve)
Preparation time: 20 minutes
Cooking time: 1 hour 40 minutes

2 small aubergines, cut into 2cm cubes *24 cals*

1-cal cooking spray

400g lamb shoulder, cut into 3cm cubes, seasoned well with salt and pepper *720 cals*

2 red onions, peeled and finely sliced *76 cals*

2 cloves garlic, finely chopped *8 cals*

2 tsp ground cumin *10 cals*

400g tin chopped tomatoes *72 cals*

2 sprigs fresh rosemary

2 tsp balsamic vinegar *3–10 cals*

4 tbsp fat-free natural yoghurt *32 cals*

2 tbsp finely shredded fresh mint *10 cals*

salt and pepper

rice, couscous or steamed green vegetables, to serve (optional)

1. Heat the oven to 200°C/400°F/Gas mark 6. Scatter the aubergine cubes in a shallow roasting tray, spray with a little 1-cal cooking spray and season well with salt and pepper. Roast for 15–20 minutes, until golden brown all over. Remove from the oven and set aside.

2. Meanwhile, spray a little cooking spray in a large heavy-bottomed flameproof casserole pan (with a lid). Heat over a medium heat and fry the lamb cubes in batches for 4–5 minutes, until golden all over. Remove from the pan and set aside.

3. Spray the pan with a little more cooking spray and then add the onions, season with salt and pepper and fry for 4–5 minutes, until softened. Add the garlic and cumin and fry for a further minute.

4. Return the cooked lamb to the pan with the tomatoes, rosemary and vinegar. Bring to the boil, then cover with the lid and simmer in the oven for 1 hour.

5. Stir in the cooked aubergine, cover with the lid again and cook for another 30 minutes in the oven.

6. In a small bowl, mix together the yoghurt and mint and season with salt and pepper.

7. To serve, divide the stew between bowls and serve with rice, couscous or steamed green vegetables and a dollop of the minty yoghurt.

THAI PRAWN SKEWERS WITH GRIDDLED COURGETTE, PEA AND MINT SALAD

This is one of the most photogenic dishes you'll ever make – and it tastes every bit as good as it looks! Prawns are a great choice on a Fast Day, and this is a glorious way to use them.

Serves 2
Calories per serving: 233
Preparation time: 20 minutes, plus marinating
Cooking time: 15 minutes

  200g large raw king prawns *140 cals*
  2 tsp lemon grass paste *8 cals*
  1 red chilli, deseeded and finely chopped *4–8 cals*
  3 tbsp chopped fresh Thai or normal basil leaves *15 cals*
  1 tsp extra-light olive oil *45 cals*
  1-cal cooking spray
  2 courgettes, cut into thin ribbons using a vegtable peeler
     68 cals
  100g frozen peas *70 cals*
  150g frozen baby broad beans *100 cals*
  zest of ½ lemon and squeeze of juice *5 cals*
  2 tbsp chopped fresh mint leaves *10 cals*
  salt and pepper

1. Place the prawns in a small bowl. Add the lemon grass paste, half the chopped chilli and the chopped basil. Spray with a little 1-cal cooking spray, season well with salt and pepper and leave to marinate for at least 10 minutes. Thread the prawns onto skewers and set aside while you prepare

the salad.

2. Heat a griddle pan until smoking hot. Spray the courgette ribbons with a little 1-cal cooking spray, season well and griddle for 1–2 minutes on each side. Repeat until all the courgette ribbons are griddled and then place in a serving bowl.

3. Blanch the peas and broad beans in boiling water for 3 minutes, then refresh/dip in cold water to stop them cooking further. (If you have time, slip the tougher outer skins off the broad beans.)

4. Add the peas and beans to the griddled courgette. Sprinkle over the lemon zest and juice, olive oil, the rest of the chopped chilli and the mint.

5. Preheat the grill to high. Place the prawn skewers on a non-stick baking sheet. Grill the prawns for 2 minutes on each side, until just charred and cooked through.

6. Serve the hot prawn skewers with the courgette salad on the side.

LEMON AND ASPARAGUS RISOTTO

Risottos are like a needy but brilliant celebrity: give them enough attention and they will reward you with star quality. This zesty dish doesn't like to be left alone, but there's a certain satisfaction as you add the stock and see the grains of rice plump up perfectly. It's a fantastic dish for family or friends to share. Serve it with garlic bread for them and a salad for you. You can use whatever ingredients you like: fresh peas and baby leeks in spring, cubes of butternut squash in autumn. Or dried and fresh mushrooms *anytime*.

Serves 4
Calories per serving: 308 (without Parmesan)
Preparation time: 15 minutes
Cooking time: 35 minutes

1-cal cooking spray
1 onion, peeled and finely chopped *38 cals*
2 sticks celery, finely chopped *12 cals*
2 cloves garlic, finely chopped *8 cals*
small handful fresh lemon thyme leaves or normal thyme leaves
     5 cals
300g Arborio rice *1,020 cals*
125ml white wine 83 cals
700ml hot fresh vegetable stock *20 cals*
100g asparagus, woody ends removed, chopped (tips
     reserved) *27 cals*
grated zest and juice 1 lemon *19 cals*
20g Parmesan cheese, freshly grated (optional) *84 cals*

1. Spray a little 1-cal cooking spray in a large heavy-based non-stick saucepan and heat over a medium heat. Add the onion and celery and fry for 2–3 minutes, until softened but not coloured. Add the garlic and fry for another minute.

2. Add the thyme and rice and stir for 2 minutes. Turn up the heat, pour in the wine and leave to bubble for a few minutes to cook off the alcohol.

3. Add the chopped asparagus (reserving the tips to add at the end). Add the hot stock, a ladleful at a time, waiting until each one is absorbed before adding the next. When the rice is almost cooked but still has a little bite to it, stir in the asparagus tips, lemon zest and juice. Cook for 3 minutes, stirring occasionally, so it doesn't stick. Serve scattered with the Parmesan, if using.

CORIANDER, LIME AND CHILLI PRAWN PASTA

This pasta* dish is prawn perfection, although you can easily vary the flavours to suit your taste or what you have fresh. Try using lemons instead of limes, and fresh basil or parsley instead of coriander.

*Yes! Pasta on a Fast Day! This recipe uses the wholewheat kind, so it keeps you full for longer. It's a great option for serving to the family, and if you want to cut calories, a veggie version would use two thinly sliced, griddled courgettes (cooked for 1–2 minutes on each side) and reduces the calories to 377 (see pages 321–322).

Serves 4
Calories per serving: 440
Preparation time: 10 minutes, plus marinating
Cooking time: 10 minutes

   400g cooked peeled king prawns *280 cals*
   finely grated zest and juice 1 lime *10 cals*
   1 red chilli, deseeded and finely chopped *4–8 cals*
   3 tbsp lemon-infused olive oil or light olive oil *405 cals*
   300g wholewheat spaghetti *990 cals*
   300g cherry tomatoes, halved *60 cals*
   large handful fresh coriander leaves, chopped *10 cals*
   salt and pepper

1. Place the prawns, lime zest and juice, chopped chilli and lemon oil in a small bowl and leave to marinate for at least 10 minutes.

2. Meanwhile, cook the pasta in a pan of salted boiling wateraccording to the packet instructions. Drain (reserving a cupful of the cooking water) and set aside.

3. Add the chopped tomatoes to the hot drained pasta with a little of the cooking water and warm through for 1–2 minutes over a medium heat. Stir in the marinated prawns and chopped coriander and warm through for 1–2 minutes. Add the cooked spaghetti and season well with salt and pepper.

HOT SMOKED SALMON AND WATERCRESS LINGUINI

A really luxurious treat for one if you've fasted all day and want to savour your calories in a single and fast, Fast Day dinner!

Serves 1
Calories per serving: 464
Preparation time: 10 minutes
Cooking time: 10 minutes

  90g linguini *317 cals*
  50g watercress *13 cals*
  grated zest of ½ lemon and a squeeze of juice *4 cals*
  2 tbsp natural virtually fat-free fromage frais *15 cals*
  50g hot smoked salmon flakes *115 cals*
  salt and pepper

1. Cook the linguini in a large pan of boiling salted water according to the packet instructions. Drain (reserving a cupful of the cooking water), return to the pan and set aside.

2. Place half the watercress, the lemon zest and a squeeze of juice, and the fromage frais in a small blender. Season with salt and pepper and blend together until smooth.

3. Stir the watercress sauce through the cooked linguini, adding a little of the reserved cooking water, as needed, to loosen the sauce. Gently mix in the reserved watercress and the smoked salmon flakes.

SPICY MEXICAN BEAN BURGERS

These cheesy, beany, spicy burgers might not be quite what you'd find on the streets of Acapulco, but they're so tasty you can forgive them a certain lack of authenticity.

You can either enjoy them with all the trimmings, or just with the halloumi for a lower calorie count. The ingredients list is quite long, but they freeze well and are really handy to have on standby for a veggie dinner.

Serves 4
Calories per serving: 244 with halloumi; 459 with burger bun, halloumi, guacamole and salad
Preparation time: 20 minutes, plus chilling
Cooking time: 20 minutes

1-cal cooking spray
½ red onion, peeled and finely chopped *19 cals*
4 spring onions, finely sliced *6 cals*
2 cloves garlic, finely chopped *8 cals*
1 large red chilli, deseeded and finely chopped *5–10 cals*
2 tsp Mexican or Cajun spice mix *10 cals*
1½ x 400g tins mixed beans, drained and rinsed *360 cals*
1 egg, beaten *78 cals*
50g fresh breadcrumbs *134 cals*
2 tbsp chopped fresh coriander leaves *10 cals*
juice of ½ lime *6 cals*
75g low-fat feta cheese, crumbled *135 cals*
80g reduced-fat halloumi cheese *204 cals*
salt and pepper

optional extras per burger

1 toasted seeded granary burger bun *180 cals per bun*
1 tbsp low-fat guacamole *17 cals*
10g rocket leaves *2 cals*
1 tomato, sliced *16 cals*

1. Spray a non-stick frying pan with a little 1-cal cooking spray. Add the onion and spring onions, season with salt and pepper and fry over a low heat for about 5 minutes, until softened but not coloured.

2. Add the garlic, chilli and Cajun spice, then fry for 2–3 minutes. Tip into a bowl, add the beans and roughly mash.

3. Leave to cool slightly, then add the egg, breadcrumbs, coriander and lime juice. Season well, then mix to combine. Gently stir in the crumbled feta.

4. Wet your hands lightly, then shape the mixture into 4 large patties. Chill in the fridge for 20 minutes to firm up.

5. Preheat the grill to medium. Spray a little more cooking spray in a grill-proof frying pan and heat over a medium heat. Add the burgers and fry for 3–4 minutes on each side, until golden brown. Top each burger with a slice of halloumi, then cook under the grill for 3–4 minutes, until the cheese is bubbling and melted.

6. Serve in toasted buns topped with guacamole, rocket leaves and sliced tomatoes, if desired.

How to freeze: Place the uncooked burgers on a baking sheet lined with non-stick baking paper. Freeze until they are solid, then pack into a freezer-proof plastic container and freeze for up to 3 months. You can cook the burgers from frozen; preheat the oven to 200°C/400°F/Gas mark 6 and preheat a baking sheet. Place the burgers on the hot baking sheet and spray with 1-cal cooking spray on both sides. Cover loosely with foil and bake for 30 minutes, turning halfway through. Preheat the grill to medium. Remove the foil, cover each burger with a slice of cheese and grill for 3–4 minutes, until the cheese is melted and bubbling.

5:2 Know–How

HOLIDAYS AND CELEBRATIONS

Once you've worked out your 5:2 routine, it's easy to stay on track. One of the advantages of 5:2 is that you can usually plan your week to allow for a big party or weekend away, for example. But longer holidays or work conferences with giant breakfast buffets, can present more of a challenge. Here are a few ideas and tips for keeping the balance:

- **Fast when you're actually travelling** so you can eat when you arrive. Aeroplane meals are rarely noted for their gourmet taste, so why not fast on the plane, bus or train, and then when you get to your destination, you're ready to try the local delights.

- **Eat less *before and after* your holiday.** I've switched to 4:3 for the week before and after a holiday, so that I don't feel bad about not sticking to 5:2 while I'm away. Or you could try two consecutive Fast Days before and after.

- **Self-catering holidays** can be the best way to try the regional cuisine and shop like a local. Plus you don't feel obliged to eat the hotel buffet meals just because you've already paid for them.

- **No one has to know** you're on a diet. With 5:2, some of us skip breakfast or lunch, and no one cares unless you make a big deal out of it!

- **Make a new routine.** It's the lack of routine on holiday that can knock you off course, so decide what suits: maybe miss breakfast or lunch, but then don't worry about what you eat at your other meals. And if you fancy that ice cream, or pastry, then why not? You're on holiday!

- **Don't weigh yourself immediately after a holiday.** Why make yourself feel bad? I know I usually put on a little weight but with 5:2 it'll be gone again soon.

- **Hotel or conference buffets are dangerous.** Research shows that we generally choose far more from a self-service buffet than we'd ever eat normally. Focus on salads and soups, eat slowly, and if you do want variety, choose very small portions of each dish.

- **Remember this is a way of life, not a punishment,** so enjoy your time off. Guilt isn't a part of 5:2. The flexibility means you can get back to your normal life next week, with lots of great memories from your holiday or celebration.

CHAPTER EIGHT

5:2 Treats

DELICIOUS DESSERTS AND DRINKS

I admit it: I have a sweet tooth. As well as a cheese tooth. And a savoury tooth. And a red-wine tooth . . . not to mention a fondness for martinis!

The idea of putting treats, sweets and cocktails in a 'diet' cookbook might seem unusual, but you've probably realised by now that this is *not* your standard diet book. I don't think desserts are essential on Fast Days, but you can easily plan for them if you choose wisely – maybe if you're having a family meal or midweek celebration. In some desserts, sweeteners can dramatically cut calories but I've always included sugar quantities too, if you prefer to avoid artificial sweeteners.

As for alcohol, obviously it's a waste of calories to drink on a Fast Day. But it doesn't mean I haven't done it. The occasional small glass of red wine or a gin and Slimline tonic, won't undo all your good work. Two, on the other hand, will probably send your willpower packing. That's why there are plenty of ideas here for yummy hot and cold drinks that will distract you from any hunger pangs, keep you hydrated and refresh the parts other diets can't reach!

RECICES

RECIPES

EMMA'S JAFFA CAKE CHOCOLATE MOUSSE

CINNAMON AND VANILLA POACHED PEARS

ELDERFLOWER JELLIES WITH BLUEBERRIES, MINT AND RASPBERRIES

STRAWBERRY AND BASIL GRANITA

FAST DAY TRIFLE TREATS

HOT DRINKS

COLD DRINKS

COCKTAILS FOR FEAST AND FAST DAYS

5:2 Lives

EMMA'S FAMILY FEASTS

'It doesn't feel like a life sentence, it feels like freedom.'

Emma Hasson from Derry in Northern Ireland, found it hard to focus on weight loss with young children to care for. It was particularly tough after the birth of her fourth child in 2012.

'After I had my third child, I lost 44.5kg (98 lb) doing Weight Watchers, then promptly got pregnant and put 19kg (42 lb) on after the baby was born in 2012. I'd managed to lose 6.5kg (14 lb) of the baby weight prior to starting 5:2 but I was getting so fed up counting points. I was unmotivated and felt I was getting nowhere fast. I desperately needed a shake-up and a change and something that I could stick to long term.'

And it turns out that fasting was exactly the shake-up she needed. Emma, who is 31, was inspired by her mother's success; she had lost 12.5kg (28 lb) in six months after watching the BBC *Horizon* documentary.

'5:2 seemed to me like it was a much more liveable plan than forever having to track and count – and my mother's weight loss encouraged me to give it a try. I started in January 2013 and after less than two months, I've lost 5kg (11 lb). I've gone from a BMI of 26 to one just in the healthy range at 24.9. I still have a way to go to get back to my goal weight, but I am making progress and don't feel deprived. It has been very nice to see my body fat percentage dropping to a healthy level.'

Emma's recipe blog, www.eenymeenymeeats.wordpress. com, is packed with original recipes and ideas, although with titles like Chorizo and Thyme Fougasse Bread, Ultimate Cauliflower Cheese and Profiteroles with Mars Bar Ganache, it's fair to say they're not *all* Fast Day friendly . . .

Emma's Fast Day Diary

Breakfast is tea with sweetener. I drink sparkling mineral water throughout the day. At around 4 p.m., I'll usually crack and have some butternut squash soup for around 50 calories. I save the majority of my calories for my evening meal. I try to make things that I can feed the whole family like ratatouille, vegetable chilli or a prawn stir-fry. I bulk out their meals with rice, noodles or pasta so it's easily adaptable to fit in with normal family life.

Feast Day Secrets

I try to be sensible on my Feast Days. Breakfast is typically porridge or chopped fruit with yoghurt and a sprinkling of granola. Lunch is a sandwich or soup. I snack on fruit. I try to have a healthy evening meal; often it's a stir-fry, although sometimes it's a much more indulgent shepherd's pie with cheesy mash topping. If I meet a friend for coffee during the week I don't worry about having a little slice of cake along with it, or enjoying a glass of wine if I can ever find a willing babysitter!

Favourite Foods

I have a sweet tooth and so cakes, desserts and chocolate have always been my downfall. I'm a keen baker and I'm frequently asked to make desserts or birthday cakes for others.

Fast Day Top Tip

- Stay flexible and remember the Scarlett O'Hara adage, 'after all, tomorrow is another day.' I don't have set Fasting Days, I move them around according to my schedule that week.

The Best Thing About 5:2

The flexibility is fantastic. I love that it doesn't feel like a life sentence, it feels like freedom.

EMMA'S JAFFA CAKE CHOCOLATE MOUSSE

Emma says: 'This mousse is just low enough in calories to work perfectly on a Fast Day if you've been very good all day but just need something sweet. It's also a yummy guilt-free dessert at any time.'

Serves 6
Calories per serving: 152
Preparation time: 15 minutes
Cooking time: 10–12 minutes, plus setting time

For the jelly

1 sachet sugar-free orange jelly *34 cals*
1 tbsp reduced-sugar orange marmalade *25 cals*
275ml boiling water

For the sponge

1-cal cooking spray
40g caster sugar *158 cals*
2 whole eggs *156 cals*
40g plain white flour *134 cals*

For the topping

65g orange-flavoured dark chocolate (e.g. Lindt Intense Orange) *325 cals*
2 egg whites in a spotlessly clean bowl *32 cals*
1 tsp caster sugar *15 cals*
4 tbsp fat-free fromage frais *30 cals*

1. Place the contents of the jelly sachet in a jug with the marmalade. Add the boiling water and stir until the jelly and marmalade have both dissolved. Make up to 570ml with cold water, following the packet instructions. Leave to cool a little.

2. Line a 20cm round cake tin with cling film. Pour in the cooled jelly. Allow to cool completely before putting in the fridge to set for up to 2 hours, or overnight.

3. Preheat the oven to 180°C/350°F/Gas mark 4. Spray a six-hole muffin tin with 1-cal cooking spray. Prepare a bain-marie by bringing a large saucepan of water to the boil, reducing to a simmer and placing a heat-proof bowl in the pan so it sits on top of the water.

4. Put the sugar and the two whole eggs in the bowl and beat with a whisk for about 5 minutes, until light and fluffy and a trail will hold its shape.

5. Add the flour and continue to mix until a thick batter forms. Half fill the holes in the muffin tin with the batter. Cook in the oven for about 10–12 minutes, until light golden and springy to the touch. Remove from the oven and allow to cool in the tin.

6. When the sponge is cool, remove from the tin and place each one in the bottom of a small ramekin. Cut circles the size of the sponge discs from the set jelly and carefully place on top of the sponge.

7. To make the topping, melt the chocolate over a pan of simmering water (don't allow the bowl to touch the water) or in the microwave. Remove from the heat and allow to cool for about 5 minutes.

8. Whisk the whites until firm, add the sugar and then whisk again until firm and stiff peaks form.

9. When the chocolate has cooled, add the fromage frais and mix to combine until glossy.

10. Finally, with a metal spoon, fold the egg whites carefully into the chocolate mixture, trying to retain as much air as possible so it's fluffy. Spoon the mousse on top of the jelly and sponge, cover with cling film and put into the fridge to set for at least 4 hours.

NB: because this dish contains uncooked egg whites, it's not suitable for pregnant women.

Kate's note: this is the perfect example of how you can have your (chocolate) cake and eat it on 5:2. It takes a little extra effort, but is ideal for a meal for family and friends: no one would know I was fasting! Next time, I'm going to try making it with raspberry jelly and a bar of chocolate with added raspberry chunks for a berry chocolate mousse!

CINNAMON AND VANILLA POACHED PEARS

If there was an award for the prettiest low-calorie pudding, there'd be a battle between these pears and the Elderflower Jellies (see pages 276–277). The syrupy sauce is aromatic and just sweet enough – although if you can 'afford' the calories, then a tablespoon of half-fat crème fraîche is the perfect contrast. Use medium-sized Comice, Green Williams or Rocha pears.

Serves 4
Calories per serving: 155 with crème fraîche, 129 without
Preparation time: 15 minutes
Cooking time: 20–30 minutes

1 vanilla pod, halved
1 cinnamon stick
500ml red grape juice *315 cals*
100ml water
4 ripe pears, peeled but kept whole with the stalk intact
    200–360 cals
4 tbsp half-fat crème fraîche, to serve (optional) *104 cals*

1. Place the vanilla pod, cinnamon stick, grape juice and the water in a large saucepan. Place over a low heat and bring to the boil.

2. Carefully lower the pears into the liquid, bring back to the boil, and then turn down the heat so that it is just simmering. Cover with a lid and poach the pears for 20–30 minutes, turning occasionally to make sure they are evenly poached.

3. The pears are ready when a cocktail stick can easily be inserted into the pears and they are tender all the way through. When tender, carefully remove the pears from the pan and place in a serving dish. Return the pan to the heat and bubble the sauce over a high heat for 5–10 minutes, until it is syrupy. Pour the sauce over the pears and leave to cool. Serve warm or cold with a small spoonful of half fat crème fraîche, if using.

ELDERFLOWER JELLIES WITH BLUEBERRIES, RASPBERRIES AND MINT

Gorgeous to look at, even better to eat! The elderflower gives a sophisticated flavour that's not overpowering, and the fruits look like little jewels in the individual serving glasses. Impress family or friends – or save them all for yourself (they keep for up to four days in the fridge!).

If you're happy using sweeteners, then you can get a much lower calorie count. I've tried these with three different kinds of sweetener – Splenda®, Xylitol and a stevia-based baking blend. All gain excellent results. Just make sure to follow the instructions on the pack as the quantities are different to sugar. Splenda®, for example, substitutes volume but *not* weight, as it weighs very little.

You can cut the chilling time down if, like me, you're not a perfectionist and don't mind some of the fruit floating nearer the top. Just divide all the jelly between all the glasses on top of the fruit and chill for 2 hours. N.B. Gelatin is not suitable for vegetarians but you can use seaweed-based agar-agar; make sure you follow the instructions as it works differently.

Serves 4
Calories per serving: 102
Preparation time: 10 minutes, plus chilling
Cooking time: 5 minutes

5 leaves gelatin *15 cals*

75g caster sugar *297 cals* or equivalent sweeteners (for
example, 5 tbsp Splenda®, *30 cals*, or granular stevia-
based sweetener, *75 cals*)

300ml water

3 tbsp elderflower cordial *46 cals*

150g mixed raspberries and blueberries, plus extra to serve
65 cals

small bunch fresh mint leaves

1. Soak the gelatin leaves in cold water until soft. Place the sugar in a small saucepan with the water and heat over a low heat until the sugar has dissolved. Remove from the heat. Squeeze out the excess water from the gelatin, add to the hot sugar water and stir until melted. Add the cordial and stir well.

2. Place a small handful of fruit and mint leaves in the bottom of 4 glasses (the tips of the mint are very pretty here), add a little of the jelly mixture and chill in the fridge for 2 hours. Set the remaining jelly aside, covered with cling film but not in the fridge – it should not set.

3. Once set, divide the rest of the jelly mix between the glasses and chill until set. Serve with extra berries and mint on the side.

Variations: Other cordials and fruit pieces will also work well. I love the Belvoir Apple and Ginger (with very slim wedges of apple and a few blackcurrants or berries), or their Raspberry and Rose drink (use rose petals from your garden as a garnish, if you haven't used pesticides). Or try Bottlegreen's Lime and Coconut with slices of kiwi. It's such an adaptable recipe! Do check the calories, as fruits and cordials can vary.

STRAWBERRY AND BASIL GRANITA

So refreshing – and a lot less hassle to make than ice cream – a granita is perfect for Fast and Feast Days. If you've never had one, it's a little like a cross between a sorbet and those slush drinks I used to guzzle as a kid. Except this bursts with fresh fruit flavours – it's my new favourite summer dessert.

If you prefer to use sweeteners, then the calorie count for this will be lower – make sure you read the packet instructions, as some sweeteners, like Splenda®, use volume rather than weight as a measure. Icing sugar gives a very smooth result, partly because it affects how the ice crystals form, but you need to allow for the higher calories.

Basil goes beautifully with strawberries, giving a slight peppery accent. I've also made this with 400g of strawberries and 100g of mango: the sweetness of the mango means it needs less added sugar. Mango and raspberry with lime juice is another fabulous combination. Use whatever's in season. Blend in the same way, then add citrus juice and sugar/sweeteners to taste, making the liquid a little sharper and sweeter than you would like the end result to be, as freezing mutes the flavour of the fruit.

Serves 4
Calories per serving: 146 made with icing sugar, 56+ made
   with sweetener
Preparation time: 10 minutes, plus freezing

500g strawberries, hulled *160 cals*

100g icing sugar *395 cals* or use sweeteners

   e.g. 6-7 tablespoons of Splenda®, *36-42 cals*

juice of 1–1½ lemons (depending on sweetness of the
   strawberries) *19 cals*

20g fresh basil leaves, plus extra to garnish *10 cals*

1. Place the hulled strawberries in a blender, add the icing sugar, the juice of 1 lemon and the basil leaves. Blend until smooth, then taste and then add more lemon juice until it tastes a little too sharp and a little too sweet. It will have a subtler taste once it has been frozen.

2. Pass through a sieve and discard the seeds and big bits of basil.

3. Tip into a shallow freezer-proof container and freeze for 2 hours, or until the sides are frozen but the middle is still not completely frozen. Scrape with a fork to break up the ice crystals and then freeze again for another hour. Scrape once more to break up the crystals and then freeze until ready to serve.

4. Depending on how hard it's frozen, you may need to move the granita from the freezer to the fridge 15 minutes before serving to allow it to soften slightly. Scrape the surface with a fork to make shards. Spoon into bowls and serve immediately garnished with the smallest basil leaves.

Fast Day Trifle Treats

Presentation makes a big difference to how food tastes. When I did a two-day Cooking with Chocolate course at the Espai Sucre Restaurant/School in Barcelona (are you impressed? I am still quite proud of myself, especially as the course was in Spanish!), one of my favourite things to do was to create little individual potted desserts in glasses or *vasos*, like trifles. I thought that recreating those, but using Fast-friendly ingredients, would elevate a quick pud to more of a treat.

For the most impact, you need at least three layers: something creamy, something crunchy and something fruity. Of course, you can do the same on Feast Days using more indulgent ingredients.

To make your 'trifles', layer your chosen ingredients in a narrow drinking glass or the free ramekins you get with a ready-made dessert. Use half of the ingredients for each layer, so you end up with six layers in total, or in a shallower pot, just use one layer in a ramekin. Then add your choice of final topping ingredient and eat immediately, or chill in the fridge. The quantities listed are enough to make 1 serving, with 2 layers of each ingredient.

Layer 1: creamy	Layer 2: crunchy	Layer 3: fruity	Final topping
(Use 2 tbsp or 30ml/g)	(Use 1 tbsp or 15g, unless otherwise stated)	(50g, unless otherwise stated)	
Ricotta cheese (*40 cals*)	Flaked almonds (*94.5 cals*)	Sliced strawberries (*16 cals*) with ½ tsp balsamic vinegar (really!) or 2 twists black pepper (optional) (*5 cals*)	Dusting of cocoa powder (*2.5–5 cals*)
Half-fat crème fraîche (*52 cals*)	2 crumbled amaretti biscuits (*70 cals*)	Fresh or thawed frozen raspberries or blueberries (*19 or 28 cals*)	3 mint leaves
Fat-free Greek yoghurt (*16 cals*)	Chopped toasted hazelnuts (*100 cals*)	25g blackberries crushed or lightly stewed with ½ chopped dessert apple (*57.5 cals*)	Lemon or orange zest
Coconut (dairy free) yoghurt (*50 cals*)	Vanilla Granola (*see pages 50–51, 69 cals*)	Half a small banana (*45 cals*)	Sprinkling of ground ginger/sliced fresh ginger
Chocolate- or toffee-flavoured yoghurt e.g. Muller Light Chocolate Orange (*15–16.5 cals*)	Shelled pistachio nuts, roughly crushed (*89 cals*)	1 segmented orange with a few drops of orange flower water (optional) (*70 cals*)	A few pomegranate seeds (*5 cals*)

Quark/fromage blanc/fat-free fromage frais (*21 cals*)	1 small ginger nut biscuit, crumbled (*40 cals*)	Stewed rhubarb — add a little sweetener or ½ tsp clear honey for sweetness (*15 cals*)	A single perfect cherry (*5 cals*)
Custard-style diet yoghurt (*33–47 cals*)	1 sponge finger/boudoir biscuit (*23 cals*)	45g pineapple chunks with 1 tsp passion fruit (*27.5 cals*)	Passion fruit seeds (*5 cals*)
Low-cal rice pudding (*20 cals*)	1 shop-bought meringue, crumbled (only if serving immediately or the sugar will melt into creamy layer) (*50 cals*)	Medium peach or nectarine, sliced or grilled then sliced (*50 cals*)	A few shavings from bar of 70% dark chocolate (*10 cals*)

Hot Drinks

After one of the toughest winters in years, I'm convinced that the humble kettle is the key to staying on 5:2 when the weather's colder.

Our bodies tell us to eat on cold days, but if we're eating less on our Fast Days then we're generating less heat through the digestive process. But before you reach for the biscuit tin, fill the kettle. Warm mug, warm hands, warm heart . . .

The Old Faithfuls: Teas and Coffee

I love coffee and loathe tea. There, I've said it. But whether you like espresso or a builder's tea, they're a great pick-me-up. I've read up a lot on caffeine, and coffee in particular, and I think the warnings for people in normal health are exaggerated. I have several coffees a day with no apparent ill effect, and there's research suggesting coffee drinkers may have lower rates of Type 2 diabetes and dementia than those who don't drink it.

It is possible that coffee causes an insulin spike, which may be an issue on Fast Days, but for me, the benefits outweigh the downsides. If you *do* want to give up, then consider leaving it until you're used to fasting – you don't want to make life harder for yourself in those early days.

I have a Nespresso machine at home – the capsules are *not* cheap but I love the coffee they make and I'm saving money on Fast Days anyway. The aroma of brewing filter coffee or the ritual of making coffee in a French press can make the experience so much nicer. It's the same with tea. Why not invest in a teapot for one and enjoy the moment?

I don't count calories, as I take my coffee black – in theory there are still calories in black coffee but I don't bother too much. You do need to count calories if you take milk, though. Some people avoid cow's milk, as it can cause a sugar spike, which may not be helpful on Fast Days. Unsweetened almond milk, soy milk or rice milk are good alternatives.

If you like milky drinks generally, a mug of unsweetened almond milk – either heated in a pan or microwave – works out under 40 calories (compared to over 100 for skimmed cow's milk) and many people really enjoy the taste.

CHAI

Chai is the name for all sorts of mixed spice teas. You can either buy it in sachets or powders, or experiment with making your own – it's really warming. When you make your own, you can either add tea leaves, or do without tea for a caffeine-free drink. Make up a larger batch and reheat it whenever you fancy a cup during your Fast Day.

As the spices are infused, the calorie count is negligible, though do count any milk or sweeteners added.

1 mug water (or try with unsweetened almond milk, for around
   40 calories, or half milk and half water)
2 whole cloves
3 whole cardamom pods
3 whole black peppercorns
½ cinnamon stick

1 slice fresh root ginger

1 tsp black or green loose tea (optional)

½ teaspoon turmeric (optional) (I know this sounds weird but turmeric has all sorts of benefits to digestion and health. Though it will turn the drink bright orange!)

½ tsp clear honey (*10 cals*) or sweetener, to taste

1. Pour the mug of water into a small pan and add all the spices, except the turmeric and the tea, if using. If you have time, crush the spices lightly in a pestle and mortar first to help release their flavours. (You can also make a small bag from muslin to hold the spices to avoid the need to strain in step 3.)

2. Simmer gently, covered, for 30–45 minutes. After you've removed the tea from the heat, you can leave it to infuse for longer if you like, depending on how strong you'd like your tea.

3. Strain the liquid through a sieve and into a mug – you can try re-using the hard spices, but replace the ginger! If you're using turmeric, then add to the mug before straining in the tea. Add honey or artificial sweetener, to taste

Herb and fruit teas

These are *so* much nicer than the dishwatery ones of years ago. I love Twinings Mint Humbug and Three Ginger from Pukka Teas, which peps up my circulation on a cold day. I don't like liquorice but many people say it gives them a great burst of sweetness to satisfy any sugar cravings. Rooibos is another hit with many dieters. Fruity teas do sometimes contain calories, so check the label, but most are under 5 calories per serving, so they won't undo your hard fasting work. Here are a few more favourites from our forums – the names make me thirsty!

Yogi Tea: Egyptian Liquorice, Throat Comfort, Cinnamon Spice, Choco Chilli

Twinings: Blackcurrant Burst, Echinacea and Raspberry, Detox

Pukka: Liquorice and Peppermint, Three Fennel

Tea Pigs: Peppermint, Tung Ting Oolong

Clipper: Dandelion and Burdock, Lemon and Ginger

Homemade Infusions

Either prepare these in one mug and then strain into another mug through a tea strainer, or buy a long-handled infuser (Whittard do one for £5). Play around with the flavours you love from your spice rack or the fridge or try any combination of the following.

- Fennel Seeds (brilliant for bloating)

- Sliced or torn fresh mint leaves – I grow several different varieties, including apple and chocolate mint, and they all taste slightly different

- Cardamom pods, opened to release the seeds

- ¼ cinnamon stick

- Fresh ginger, sliced

- A chunk of lemon (you don't need to remove this but watch out for the pips!)

- Honey, lemon and ginger is a classic cold cure, but why save it for when you're poorly? Use 1 slice root ginger (no calories, as you don't eat it!), the juice of half a lemon, and 1 teaspoon clear honey (*20 cals*) or low-calorie sweetener. Put the ingredients in a mug and pour over boiling water. Leave to infuse, then pick out the ginger and lemon with a spoon if they get in the way of drinking pleasure!

Hot Chocolate

There's a wide range of comforting chocolatey drinks around. Most contain artificial sweeteners, which some people choose to avoid, but I think these can be just what you need when the chocolate cravings get too much. I like Options hot chocolates, but there are also branded ones from Cadbury's that get the thumbs up. Check the calorie counts – most are 30–40 calories but there are some 'indulgent' ones that come in nearer 60.

KATE'S MINI MOCHA

After extensive experimentation (!), I've refined the perfect Fast Day mocha.

- 1 sachet low-cal hot chocolate (e.g. Options Caramel, *39 cals*)
- 1 Nespresso capsule, or good-quality coffee granules/instant espresso powder
- 150ml boiling water
- 1 tbsp semi-skimmed or unsweetened almond milk (optional) *7 or 2 cals*

1. Empty the hot-chocolate powder into the bottom of a mug. Make the Nespresso and add to the hot chocolate. Choose the 'longer' version, stirring briskly with a teaspoon as it pours into the mug. Or mix the coffee granules/powder with hot chocolate and add the boiling water, stirring thoroughly.

2. Add the milk for extra creaminess. You can also divide the hot chocolate sachet into two portions to make two mochas – it will still have enough sweetness but with a stronger coffee flavour, of course.

Cold Drinks

Staying hydrated on Fast Days will help avoid 'diet' headaches, and also reduces hunger pangs – often we mistake thirst for hunger, so drinking lots of water will help. I work my way through a litre and a half bottle of sparkling water on a Fast Day – it feels more interesting than tap! Here are some additions to pep up either tap or fizzy water further:

- Juice of ½ orange or blood orange (*20 cals*)

- Juice of ½ grapefruit, freshly squeezed (around *38 cals*) (watch out if you're on certain medications including those to cut blood pressure, as grapefruit can change how the body processes the medication)

- Elderflower or other cordials. Try my suggestions, below.

If you have a strainer jug (with a lid that stops anything but liquid escaping through the pouring spout), you can add flavour without calories. Try these mixes and store in the fridge door:

- A wedge of lemon and 5 slices of cucumber

- Mint leaves and ¼ fresh apple, cut into chunks – you're not eating the apple so the calories are negligible.

- ½ lime and some sliced melon or strawberries – use the mushier ones from the bottom of the punnet, as the texture doesn't matter when you're not eating them

Diet Drinks

One of the most common questions I read on forums is: 'Can I drink diet drinks or use artificial sweeteners?'

Often, other forum members post documents and articles with claims about the damage that certain sweeteners can do to your health. Many of these are very dramatic but the evidence to support the claims can be dubious. I believe that as adults, we can make our own choices. All food additives in developed countries are thoroughly tested before they're approved – although we need to remember that things can go wrong at all levels of the food chain.

If you want to read the science, it's available online. My own choice, based on what I've read, is not to worry about the odd Diet Coke or Lemonade. I don't take sweeteners or sugars in hot drinks simply because I don't like the taste, but I do have occasional diet hot chocolate. I think it's about balance. One or two diet drinks a week is my personal limit. If you crave or overdo anything (not just diet drinks) then it's probably worth looking at the reasons why and trying to find alternatives or new routines.

Cocktails for Feast and Fast Days

Cocktail recipes? I told you 5:2 was different!

OK, so the Fast Day versions are mainly what restaurants like to call *mocktails* (which for some reason makes me think of Bunny Girls), but, as I confessed in *The 5:2 Diet Book,* I have been known to have an alcoholic drink on Fast Days . . . always within my calorie allowance, of course.

If you do like alcoholic drinks, here are some ideas for both Fast and Feast days.

Lower-Calorie Alcohol Choices

These guidelines are more for non-fasting days when you want to make lower calorie choices. Dry sparkling wines like Champagne and cava are said to be supermodels' choice with a fairly low calorie count (*90–100 cals per 125ml*) – though a single measure of low-calorie mixer is lower still. A small glass (125ml) of red wine is 85 calories and of white wine 83.

Sweet drinks, like liqueurs (and especially the cream-based ones) contain extra sugar on top of the sugar in the alcohol, and alco-pops are often ultra-sweet to suit people who aren't that keen on the taste of alcohol. On Feast Days it's up to you, but you *can* wean yourself off the sweeter drinks if you want to; our taste buds are very adaptable. Remember when you first tasted alcohol? Chances are you hated the taste, but it grew on you over time . . .

Cocktails

I am a cocktail lover, partly from watching too much *Mad Men* and partly after discovering so many great cocktail bars when we lived in Barcelona – Brighton doesn't disappoint on the mixology front either.

To tie in with colours of the 5:2 logo (which also happen to be my favourite colours), here are two sets of red and green cocktails. The alcohol-free versions mean you can still enjoy a colourful and tempting drink on Fast Days – and the stronger cocktails are perfect for when you're celebrating reaching a weight loss milestone. Cheers!

Red Drinks

At home, our favourite martini is a Cosmopolitan, made famous by the *Sex and the City* girls. It's the drink my partner, Richard, makes when we're celebrating, or before going out for a big night! Yes, it's boozy and one for Feast Days. But there's a Fast Day version, too.

All measures are 25ml unless otherwise stated and all drinks serve 1.

FEAST DAY: RICHARD'S COSMO

Calories per cocktail: 224

2 measures vodka *112 cals*

1 measure triple sec (e.g. Cointreau) *85 cals*

squeeze fresh lime juice *2 cals*

2 measures cranberry juice *25 cals*

(Adjust up for more than one person – or down for less alcohol, but the proportions stay the same!)

orange peel, to garnish

1. Put all ingredients in a cocktail shaker with lots of ice. Shake well (Richard says the sound changes when you've shaken thoroughly to more of a 'thump').

2. Strain into a martini glass. Garnish with a strip of orange peel that you've 'flamed' by holding next to a lit match until the oils spit a little and release their aroma.

FAST DAY: KATE'S COSMOPO-LIGHT-AN

Calories per mocktail: 23

2 measures light cranberry juice *4 cals*

squeeze of fresh lime juice *2 cals*

2 measures fresh orange juice or 1 measure fresh orange and 1 measure grapefruit *18 cals or 17 cals*

orange peel, to garnish

1. Prepare in exactly the same way as a normal Cosmo including the garnish! If you want a little alcohol, 1 measure of vodka is 56 calories.

Green Drinks

Our favourite bar in Barcelona used to be called Gimlet. It really did make you feel like Don Draper or Joan Harris from *Mad Men,* with the polished wood bar, the even more polished bar staff and the dreadful silence if you so much as whispered the word Cosmopolitan – any drink invented post-1960 was cocktail-non-grata. It's changed its name to Cocktail Bar Juanra Falces but the fearsomely strong drinks are the same!

FEAST DAY: GIMLET

A knockout, although too many will also knock you out.

Calories per cocktail: 87

25ml measure gin (I like Hendrick's but use your favourite brand) about *56 cals*
25ml measure lime cordial *31 cals*
cocktail cherry, to serve

1. Shake together with ice. Strain. Serve with a cocktail cherry (green and almost red!).

FAST DAY: NOJITO

Just like a Mojito. But without the sugar, or the alcohol (well, you can have some if you insist).

Calories per mocktail: 30 (or 88 with a 25ml measure of white rum)

> ½ teaspoon Truvia baking blend or other granular sweetener *5 cals*
> 1 lime, quartered, plus extra to garnish *20 cals*
> 8 fresh mint leaves, plus extra to garnish *5 cals*
> crushed ice
> 25ml white rum e.g. Bacardi (optional) *58 cals*
> 300ml soda water

1. Pound or 'muddle' the sweetener, lime quarters and half the mint in a pestle and mortar to release the flavours.

2. Place crushed ice in a tall glass, to a quarter of the height. Add the muddled fruits and whole mint leaves and the rum, if using. Top with more ice, then fill to the top with soda water. Garnish with a slice of lime and a mint leaf.

5:2 Know-How

5:2 FOR LIFE

5:2 is the first 'diet' I've actually believed I can stick to for life – in fact, I actively *want* to stay on this plan, because of the health benefits and the freedom it offers me. So, once you've reached your goal weight, here are some ideas for staying on track permanently.

6:1 – a single Fast Day per week is a good choice for many people who are doing intermittent calorie restriction for health reasons. Sticking to at least one Fast Day each week mean our bodies still get a break. It also keeps us aware of the right amount to eat the rest of the time.

Staying flexible. Of course, the flexibility of this approach also means that we're able to go back up to two days a week before or after holidays, or if we sense the weight creeping back on.

Weighing In? It's worth thinking about how you'll monitor your weight. Many of us have mixed feelings about the scales, especially as your weight can vary so much day by day, but equally it's easy to let weight creep back on. So whether you decide to weigh yourself once a week or once a fortnight, or choose to monitor your weight with a tape measure or the pair of jeans that fit perfectly at your ideal size, it's good to have a regular check-in so that all your work to lose the weight won't be in vain. Weight creeps on gradually so nip it in the bud before it gets out of control.

Beware of bigger portions! Fast Days should keep us aware of portion sizes, which can creep back up after a weight-loss success on other plans, with us barely noticing. As I mentioned in How to 5:2 (see pages 9–32), after we lose weight, our calorie needs also reduce, because we've less weight to move around. So if you go back to your 'old ways', the weight will go back on. Recording what you eat on Fast Days, even if it's just in a notebook, will maintain an awareness of good habits.

Research for the future. Though fasting is as old as mankind itself, the interest in this approach for health and weight loss is growing, as is the research. At the moment, we don't have all the answers about how it will work long term, or the best way to maximise benefits. So staying in touch – whether it's through a forum, Facebook group, or books – makes sense. See the Tool Kit section for resources (see pages 352–353).

CHAPTER NINE

5:2 Extras

SAUCES, DRESSINGS AND SWAPS

It's a tough job being in the background. One of my more unusual career moves was being an extra or 'supporting artiste' for movies and television. Unnoticed, mainly, and not very glamorous, but boy, if you get it wrong, you'll stand out for all the wrong reasons. While if you get it right, you enhance the production by adding flavour and pizzazz.

So it is with the dishes in this chapter. A tomato sauce might not set the world on fire, but it can act as the backdrop for so many great dishes. Likewise, a good salad dressing will give the humble lettuce leaf star billing.

Plus, we've lots of suggestions for ways to enhance a special sauce or fab main, or to make your soups even tastier. The nominations are in for best supporting recipe – which one will you choose?

RECITES

SIMONE'S CAULIFLOWER RICE

SAUCES, SALSAS AND SALAD DRESSINGS

THE ONLY TOMATO SAUCE YOU'LL EVER NEED
PLUS
MEXICAN, HOT ITALIAN, WARMING INDIAN, SWEET SPANISH PAPRIKA

FRUITY AND FRESH SALSA

SMOKY AND PEPPERY SALSA

DRESSINGS AND DIPS

MAGICAL STOCKS

PASTA AND POTATO SWAPS

5:2 Lives

SIMONE'S WEDDING

'It's made me re-examine my relationship with food – and take control of my body.'

As she prepares for her summer wedding, Simone Baker can look back on an amazing year – she's lost 15.5kg (34 lb) in weight and also started exercising again, despite long-standing disabilities.

Simone's weight issues began in childhood. Her mother had taken the drug Thalidomide during pregnancy, which affected Simone's development.

'I have always been overweight, since the age of nine. My weight continued to increase once I got married and had my daughter, Lois. Then I had a really bad car crash in 2002 and sustained a serious injury that further reduced my already very limited mobility.'

The accident meant Simone, from Reading in Berkshire, had to stop work, needed to use a wheelchair outside the house and could no longer exercise. It was a vicious circle, and the weight piled on. In February 2012, Simone decided enough was enough.

'At the age of 50 it was time to take control of my body and what I was unintentionally doing to it. I didn't fancy having high blood pressure, diabetes or any other weight-induced illnesses on top of my existing physical problems.'

It wasn't the first time Simone had tried to lose weight. 'I'd had other (failed) attempts at losing weight by attending diet classes, but I'd get fed up or bored and would put all the weight back on and some more!'

This time, Simone began logging her calories on an online weight-loss website and, at first, the plan worked; Simone's a really keen cook and she created tasty, lower-calorie dishes. But by autumn, she was struggling to stay under her recommended 1,300 calories per day.

Then she heard about 5:2. The flexibility was exactly what she needed, and by March 2013, she'd gone from a size 24 to a size 18. Weight loss is only part of the story.

'I've changed from doing no exercise, to over an hour a day, including walking for 25 minutes on a treadmill. Whilst I will always need a wheelchair for distances, I am now much more mobile. I also used to get occasional asthma, and I no longer do. The ankle that I injured in the accident was previously swollen and painful and has been like that for ten years, but the exercise has reduced the pain and isn't swollen at all now. My physio has been incredulous at the difference!'

Simone aims to be 6.7kg (147 lb) in time for her wedding to Andy in August. 'My final goal weight is 60kg (133 lb), but once
I reach that, I see 5:2 as being a way to maintain it long term.'

Simone's Fast Day Diary

I either save all my calories for one meal at the end of the day, at around 5 p.m., or I have a very low-calorie meal at midday (usually homemade soup or a salad for around 150–200 calories) and the remainder of my calories for my evening meal. I try to avoid teas and coffees and stick to fruit tea and water. I exercise on Fast Days and actually enjoy my exercise more than on non-Fast Days!

Feast Day Secrets

Breakfast on a Feast Day is usually cereal (muesli, porridge or bran flakes) with almond milk and 10g of Chia Seeds. Lunch is either homemade soup or salad with chicken, ham, smoked salmon or tuna. Dinner could be anything! But it always includes lots of vegetables or salad. I love all kinds of fish, especially salmon!

I do like the odd treat. I have either a 100-calorie chocolate bar, a small glass of wine, a chocolate-covered rice cake, some Sunbite crisps, fresh mango or some fruity yoghurt (my favourite is apple and cinnamon!).

Fast Day Tips

- Choose foods that need a lot of chewing (salads!).

- Make your meals special; take time to enjoy them at a table that is properly laid, if possible with company.

Favourite Foods

I love all foods. I am lucky because I love vegetables and it really isn't any effort to make sure I have my five a day! I love a roast dinner, but tend not to have much meat but around five or six vegetables (and it has to include roast parsnips!).

The Best Thing About 5:2

I actually enjoy a day off from thinking about food. It's made me re-examine my relationship with food and come to terms with the fact that I can skip meals and feel OK.

I love that I can let the reins out over a weekend or at social events, but fasting before or after keeps me on track.

SIMONE'S CAULIFLOWER RICE

Simone says: 'This has been an absolute Godsend to my Fast Days, as 100g of cauliflower rice is only 24 calories, compared to 100g of rice being 355 calories! I even had it with Christmas dinner! Serve it in place of normal rice, mashed potatoes or pasta. It has a very mild taste, even if you don't like cauliflower. It's great with things like curries and Bolognese, as the cauliflower absorbs the flavours of the sauces you serve it with. For the calorie saving alone, this is one of my regular favourites.'

Serves 2 (or keep 1 portion covered in fridge for later that day)
Calories per portion: 16
Preparation time: 5–15 minutes
Cooking time: 5–10 minutes

½ head small cauliflower (about 130g), cut into florets
   32 cals

1. Grate or finely chop the cauliflower florets until they resemble rice grains. (The fastest way to do this is using the chopping blade or grater in a food processor, but it will result in a finer texture that's a little more like couscous. Pulse to make sure it's not over-processed.)

2. Cook on full power in the microwave for 2 minutes in a lightly covered microwavable dish (reduce to 60 seconds if using one portion's worth). Don't add water: there's already enough water in the cauliflower to stop it drying out.

3. If you don't have a microwave, steam the cauliflower pieces in a steamer (with fine holes, so the grains won't fall through) or in a sieve sat over

a pan of simmering water (cover the sieve tightly with foil to allow the cauliflower to steam) for 2 minutes. Or, stir-fry in a hot pan — with a splash of water to prevent it from sticking — for 2–3 minutes, until softened.

Kate says: I was sceptical at first but I am now a total convert. I also like to add fresh green herbs or spices when I pulse it in the food processor: a sprig of rosemary or a few chilli flakes. I'll make 4 portions at a time, store it in a plastic box and use the other portions within 24 hours. I've even tried it on my friends and they had no idea it was cauliflower!

Sauces, Salsas and Salad Dressings

The key to successful Fast Day food is keeping things fresh and interesting. Sauces, salsas and salad dressings offer maximum flavour for minimum calories: but shop-bought accompaniments can be surprisingly high in oils or sugars that can easily send you way over your Fast Day allowance.

Don't despair! There are already plenty of great recipes throughout the book for dressings and sauces you might want to try out.

Recipe	Try with	Page
Sauces		
Chunky Tomato Sauce	Anything!	140–141
Minty Yoghurt Sauce	Veggie or chicken burgers	117–118

Salsas		
Pineapple Chilli Salsa	Chicken or fish	111–112

Dressings and Dips		
Horseradish and Balsamic Dressing	Root vegetables like beetroot, or cold meats	159–160
Lemon, Honey and Hazelnut Dressing	Warm asparagus or goat's cheese	179–180
Basil Yoghurt Dressing	Little Gem, chicory and other crisp lettuces/leaves	177–178
Belinda's Zingy, Spicy Dressing	All veggies and cooked chicken	170–171
Asian Dressing (from Beef Stir-fry)	Grilled tofu, green veg	315
Waldorf Dressing	Any salad, radicchio, or finely shredded cabbage	188

Over the next few pages are some more *really* fast and easy sauces, salsas and dressings to keep your taste buds happy without ruining your Fast Days. In many cases, you can freeze or keep them in the fridge for several days to reduce the work you need to do in the kitchen.

THE ONLY TOMATO SAUCE YOU'LL EVER NEED

You can use this sauce as a base for courgette pasta (see pages 321–322), chicken dishes, and vegetable and bean soups or stews. Choose different seasonings according to what you are cooking with it. On Feast Days, splash out a little with some nice olive oil instead of 1-cal cooking spray. This freezes well or will keep in a plastic container in the fridge for up to three days. Try the variations underneath the main recipe for a twist on the classic sauce.

Serves 4
Calories per serving: 25
Preparation time: 5 minutes
Cooking time: 8 minutes

  1-cal cooking spray
  1 clove garlic, crushed or finely chopped *4 cals*
  1 tbsp balsamic vinegar (optional) *4–16 cals*
  400g tin chopped tomatoes *72 cals*
  1 tsp Marigold bouillon (or similar powdered stock) *12 cals*
  1 tsp tomato purée *3–10 cals*
  small handful fresh herbs (anything you have growing but basil,
      parsley, oregano and thyme are especially good) *5 cals*
  salt and pepper

1. Spray a medium non-stick saucepan with 3 sprays of 1-cal cooking spray. Fry the garlic over a low heat for 1–2 minutes — make sure it doesn't burn. Add a little splash of water if it sticks, and then add the balsamic vinegar, if using.

2. Add the other ingredients except the fresh herbs. Bring to the boil, then reduce to a simmer and cook for 5 minutes, stirring to stop it sticking.

3. Chop or tear the leaves and stir into the mix. Season with salt and pepper.

MEXICAN TOMATO SAUCE

To use with Huevos 'Fasteros', pages 59–60.

(around 30 calories per serving)

1. Add 1–2 finely chopped fresh jalapenos (deseeded, optional) (*4–8 cals*) or 1 teaspoon chipotle pepper paste from a jar (*4–10 cals*), plus 3–4 small spring onions (*3–8 cals*) to the pan when you fry the garlic. Leave out the balsamic vinegar and basil, but add freshcoriander leaves when you serve.

HOT ITALIAN

(40 calories per serving)

1. Use extra garlic (at least 2 cloves, *8 cals*), a chopped sweet red pepper (*40 cals*) and a finely chopped chilli pepper (*4–8 cals*) or a pinch of dried chilli flakes. Fry these together with the garlic for 3–4 minutes. Add either a teaspoon of Italian dried herbs when you add the tinned tomatoes, or stir in fresh oregano and marjoram at the end. You can experiment with tinned plum or cherry tomatoes instead of chopped, and break them up a little with a fork while simmering. I often throw in extra-ripe halved cherry tomatoes for the last couple of minutes to add texture.

WARMING SPICY INDIAN

(40 calories per serving)

1. Chop a medium onion (*38 cals*) and fry for 2–3 minutes until softened, before adding the garlic and half a teaspoon each of turmeric, cumin seeds and coriander seeds (*about 5 cals*), plus a pinch of chilli flakes for heat if you like. A pinch of garam masala stirred in near the end of cooking adds a lovely sweetness. Serve with fresh coriander leaves — and a tablespoon of fat-free Greek yoghurt is a lovely topping (*8 cals*).

SWEET SPANISH PAPRIKA

(around 40 calories per serving)

1. Add a teaspoon of smoked paprika (*5 cals*) — worth buying just for the beautiful tins — to the garlic and fry together. You can also add a chopped sweet pepper (*40 cals*) and ½ teaspoon each of ground cumin and cinnamon (*6 cals*) for a more Moroccan/north-African flavour.

2. For a sweeter flavour, add 1 tablespoon of sultanas (*42 cals*) when you add the chopped tomatoes and top with 10g flaked, toasted almonds (*63 cals*). If you add 300g cauliflower, broken into florets (*75 cals*), and half a drained 390g tin chickpeas (*135 cals*) at the same time as the garlic, you'll have yourself a tasty veggie stew!

Salsas

Adapt to suit whatever you have in the fruit bowl or fridge. Try watermelon or papaya instead of mango in the fruity salsa; sweetcorn and rinsed white beans added to the peppery salsa will make a substantial salad.

FRUITY AND FRESH SALSA

I love sweet and spicy flavours mixed together – and the colours are gorgeous too.

Serves 2
Calories per serving: 38
Preparation time: 5–10 minutes

½ small ripe mango, peeled and chopped (I have been known to cheat by dicing 100g pre-prepared mango) *55–70 cals*
2 spring onions, finely chopped *3 cals*
½ red chilli, deseeded and finely chopped (increase to whole chilli for an extra kick) *2–4 cals*
juice and zest ½ lime *10 cals*
small handful chopped fresh coriander or parsley *5 cals*
salt and pepper

1. Mix all the ingredients together in a bowl. It's that simple! Serve with fish or chicken, or with a large salad with some low-fat feta or fresh mozzarella cheese – the zingy fruit and creamy cheese are a match made in heaven.

SMOKY AND PEPPERY SALSA

The smoky flavours in this one come from grilling the sweet peppers and from chipotle peppers, which are jalapeño chillies that have been smoked and dried. You can buy the paste in jars in supermarkets, or reconstitute dried peppers the same way as dried mushrooms. But do remove the stalks and seeds before using. This makes loads – and like the previous salsa, everyone will love it (even if they've never even heard of fasting), so it's perfect for a party!

Serves 6–8
Calories per serving: 19–14
Preparation time: 10–15 minutes
Cooking time: 10–12 minutes

1 medium red pepper (or use 1 roast pepper from a jar)
    30 cals
2 ripe tomatoes 32 cals
¼ cucumber, deseeded and finely chopped 8 cals
1 small clove garlic, crushed 4 cals
juice of ½ lime 10 cals
pinch sea salt
½ tsp chipotle paste 3–10 cals
½ red onion, peeled and finely chopped 19 cals
small handful chopped fresh coriander or flat-leaf parsley 5 cals
pepper

1. Preheat the grill to medium-high. Cut the pepper in half, place on a baking sheet cut-side down and grill for 10–12 minutes, until charred.

Transfer to a bowl to cool, then remove seeds, pith and peel away the blackened skin.

2. If you have a food processor, place all ingredients except the onion and coriander in the processor and pulse until chopped but still chunky. Mix in the onions and herbs and season with pepper.

3. If you're making this by hand, chop all the veggies very finely, and mix together in a bowl. Add chopped herbs and season with pepper.

Dressings and Dips

The fastest dressing is a little balsamic or cider vinegar straight from the bottle, or half a lemon squeezed over your salad. But sometimes you want more . . .

The dips featured throughout the book can work as dressings, too, especially in sandwiches or wraps. Try the Roasted Squash Hummus or the Baba Ganoush (see pages 240 or 242). They're thicker than dressings but avoid the need for butter, keeping fillings moist and tasty!

For all the following recipes, simply put the ingredients in a clean jam jar, put the lid back on and give them a good shake. You can then keep the jar in the fridge. I did buy a plastic salad shaker, which is longer and thinner and has dressing recipes on the side (very oily, so Feast Day only!). You could even use a cocktail shaker, but wash it thoroughly afterwards, unless you fancy a garlicky Martini!

Alternatively, place the ingredients in a small bowl and whisk thoroughly until combined and smooth. Season with salt and pepper, to taste. Keep an eye on the salt content in those that already include soy sauce.

Even though these are generally lower in calories than dressing with oil alone, some still come in quite high in calories, so measure carefully and be sparing on Fast Days.

SWEET AND SOUR BALSAMIC DRESSING

This is quite runny and so good!

Makes: 150ml
Calories per teaspoon: 5

4 tbsp balsamic vinegar *20–60 cals*
1 tbsp light soy sauce *6 cals*
1 tsp Dijon mustard *5 cals*
1 tbsp clear honey *60 cals*
3 tbsp fat-free Greek yoghurt *24 cals*
1–2 tsp extra-virgin olive oil *45–90 cals*

CREAMY HERB DRESSING

Tastes so much richer than you'd believe from the calorie count!
Use less milk to make a thicker dressing.

Makes: 100ml
Calories per teaspoon: 5

50g Philadelphia Light with Garlic and Herbs (or try the Sweet
    Chilli for a different flavour) *73 cals*
1–2 tbsp finely chopped fresh herbs *5–10 cals*
2 tbsp semi-skimmed milk *14 cals*
juice of ½ lemon *4–10 cals*

WEST COUNTRY DRESSING

Very fresh-tasting, though higher in calories than the previous dressings. You can dilute the vinegar by adding 1 teaspoon of water to 2 teaspoons of vinegar if you don't like it too sharp.

Makes: about 55ml
Calories per teaspoon: 26

- 2 tbsp extra virgin olive oil *270 cals*
- 1 tbsp cider vinegar *3 cals* or dilute as above
- ½ tsp clear honey *10 cals* (if it's not sweet enough, add Truvia or other sweetener)
- ¼ tsp mustard powder (or ½ tsp wholegrain) *2–4 cals*
- juice of ½ lemon *3–10 cals*

PIQUANT ITALIAN DRESSING

The quantities are similar to the West Country version, but the garlic, chilli and red wine vinegar make this variation *bellisimo!*

Makes: about 55ml
Calories per teaspoon: 26

- 2 tbsp extra virgin olive oil *270 cals*
- 1 tbsp red wine vinegar *3–5 cals* or dilute as above
- ½ tsp clear honey *10 cals* (if it's not sweet enough, add Truvia or other sweetener

1 clove garlic, crushed *4 cals*
generous pinch chilli flakes
finely chopped fresh basil leaves

NUTTY ASIAN DRESSING

Deeply savoury and smoky; use sparingly. Great on steamed broccoli or other cooked vegetables as well as salads.

Makes: 100ml
Calories per teaspoon: 17

2 tbsp sesame oil (or 1 sesame and 1 groundnut oil) *270 cals*
4 tbsp soy sauce *24 cals*
1 clove garlic *4 cals*
¼ tsp pre-prepared ginger, finely grated *3 cals*
1 tsp toasted sesame seeds *32 cals*
finely chopped fresh coriander and basil leaves (Thai or normal)

Magical Stocks

I have a confession to make: I'd never actually made my own stock until I wrote this book. I realise this is a food crime right up there with preferring Dairy Milk to Godiva, but as a veggie, I'd never tried. Then I talked to Anna, the lovely home economist who has worked on the book with me, and asked her which kind of stock cubes she'd recommend. She was very polite, but I got the impression she'd use stock cubes over her dead body.

Suitably shamed, I've been experimenting. And wishing I'd started decades ago. Having a stockpot bubbling away makes me feel more of a domestic goddess than baking a dozen cupcakes.

One issue for us is estimating the calorie content. With veggie stock, it's less of an issue as you're controlling the fat. With chicken or beef stock, it's harder, as part of the flavour comes from the fat in the carcass or bones. Shop-bought fresh stock will be higher in calories, as it uses more fat and also additions like flour. In recipes, we have allowed 25 calories per 1 litre of vegetable stock, 30–45 for a light chicken stock and 50 calories for a litre of beef.

VERY, VERY BASIC FAST DAY VEGGIE STOCK

The liquid will keep for several days in the fridge, or freeze soup-sized portions for up to a year (you can melt them straight into the pan). Or you can freeze it in ice-cube trays, putting the cubes in a bag or box once frozen and snapping off as many as you like at a time.

This is a base recipe: you can add a couple of chopped mushrooms or just the stalks, some tomatoes, a parsnip, a clove or two of garlic or some fennel. Experiment with adding the rind from a Parmesan cheese for an extra savoury kick! Keep a stock bag/tub in the fridge or freezer and add veg peelings as you go, then tip into the stock pan when you're ready to make your stock (check nothing's gone mouldy first!).

Preparation time: 5 minutes
Cooking time: 50 minutes, plus resting

    ½ tsp olive oil
    2 onions, peeled and roughly chopped
    2 leeks, roughly chopped
    2 carrots, chopped into chunks (don't bother to peel)
    2 sticks celery, chopped into chunks
    2 fresh bay leaves
    ½ tsp peppercorns
    sprig fresh thyme
    fresh woody parsley stems

1. Heat the olive oil in a large non-stick saucepan. (I don't use 1-cal cooking spray for this, as a little 'real' fat gives flavour to stock. As a base for

Asian soups and stews, try using coconut oil.) Fry the veg for 2–3 minutes, until lightly browned.

2. Add enough water (about 1.5 litres) to cover the veggies, bring to the boil, then simmer for 30–45 minutes. Turn off the heat and leave the vegetables for as long as possible (a minimum of an hour) before straining through a sieve. Allow to cool.

CHICKEN OR MEAT STOCK

1. Add the bones from a roast chicken or meat bones along with the water, and simmer for at least 1–2 hours. Drain, cool and refrigerate/freeze as above.

2. For white chicken stock, put all the ingredients into the pan and cover with water. Bring to the boil and then reduce the heat to a simmer and cook gently for 2–3 hours, skimming frequently to remove any impurities. Use within 3 days or freeze.

FISH STOCK

1. Use the trimmings or shells from seafood or fish. Fish bones and trimmings should be rinsed well before use. This will help to ensure the stock isn't too cloudy or have any impurities. Make as the other stocks, but it will need skimming regularly with a large metal spoon. Simmer gently for about 30 minutes. Use within 3 days or freeze.

2. Be warned, fish stock can make the house whiff a bit, so use the extractor fan to the max, or you may prefer to buy this in!

Pasta and Potato Swaps

Pasta and potato present two problems on Fast Days: they're high in calories *and* carbohydrates. So first you have to have a tiny portion not to break your calorie limit. And second, the blood sugar dip after eating may make you hungry again quite quickly.

Simone's Cauliflower Rice (see pages 303–304) makes a great replacement for pasta and potato. Here are some more ideas for the days when you need something heartier than just a few rocket leaves.

Baked Sweet Potato

Sweet potatoes aren't very different in calorie terms from normal potatoes, but they offer more nutritionally and, most importantly for Fast Days, they're usually smaller so you can have a whole baked jacket. One weighing 100g is 90 calories. Bake for 35–45 minutes or microwave for 4–5 minutes. They go well with pulse dishes or with a crème fraîche topping.

Couscous

Again, in itself there's nothing low cal about couscous, but it is easy to prepare and you can control the portion size down to the last gram. It contains 94 calories per 25g dry weight, which looks like nothing but plumps up! It is good hot or cold with flavourings forked through, like spring onions, a teaspoon of raisins, sultanas or pine nuts, chopped tomatoes, toasted sesame seeds, chopped herbs, or just a splash of Worcestershire sauce or lemon juice with lots of pepper.

I've also just tried barley couscous, which has an earthier taste and is slightly lower in calories at 85 calories for 25g dry weight. It's expensive but as you only use a little on Fast Days, it's well worth trying.

COURGETTE 'PASTA'

Like Cauliflower Rice (see pages 303–304), making a pasta substitute from courgettes might seem eccentric, but on Fast Days, when every calorie counts, this is a way to make a filling side dish that can carry a sauce and increase your vegetable count.

It's one of those dishes where having a little hand-held mandolin (see page 96) can really speed things up. Or use a Y-shaped peeler.

A medium-sized courgette will serve 2 as a side dish or 1 as a main dish with sauce. The calorie count of 34 calories compares to 180 calories for a small 100g portion of fresh egg tagliatelle.

Serves 1 as a main dish
Calories per serving: 34 calories (about 37 if you use the frying method)
Preparation time: 3 minutes
Cooking time: 1–2 minutes

   1 courgette (170g) *34 cals*
   salt and pepper

1. Wash the courgette and cut off the stem and base. If you have a mandolin, set it to a medium setting, to end up with strips around 2–3mm deep. Or use a normal peeler, pressing hard so you end up with thicker slices than you would if you were simply peeling the veg. It can take a bit of practice but it is very satisfying. Cut strips running the entire length of the courgette, and move the vegetable as you slice, so that most pieces have a nice green strip on the edges.

2. Bring a small pan of salted water to a rolling boil, drop the ribbons into the water and boil for 45 seconds–1 minute, depending on how thinly they're sliced. Drain very well, and return to pan to season before serving. Or, you could fry the courgette strips in a non-stick frying pan. Spray the pan with 1-cal cooking spray and heat. Toss the ribbons in the pan and make sure they're spread across the base. Cover the pan with a lid, turn down the heat and let them cook for 1 minute before turning the ribbons over and cooking for a further minute on the other side. Remove from the heat, season to taste and serve. (I prefer this method.)

Serving Ideas

Add the juice and zest of half a lemon (*10 cals*), a few basil leaves and 20g crumbled low-fat feta cheese (*36 cals)* and lots of pepper.

This is also nice with the Mushroom Stroganoff on page 246.

It's so low in calories that you could use your own favourite pasta sauce (make sure you count the calories)

Serve at room temperature in summer with thin slices of fennel or red onion: a mix of yellow and green courgettes makes this a very pretty dish.

ZERO OR SHIRATAKI NOODLES

Shirataki noodles have become the big news for many dieters lately. They're translucent noodles from Japan, made from a form of yam and contain virtually no calories or carbs (though some have tofu which raises the calorie count a little). Shirataki means 'white waterfall' which gives you an idea of what they look like. They contain water and glucomannan, which is a kind of dietary fibre.

Some 5:2 dieters swear by them as they're filling and 'cost' so few calories from your Fast Day limit – but they are also pretty tasteless without a sauce. Or worse, they have a fishy smell due to the water they come soaked in, unless you rinse them very thoroughly.

Dry roasting them in a pan can help make them tastier – use a non-stick pan and 'fry' for a minute or two until the texture changes and they squeak!

They can be expensive, but the cheapest place will be a local Asian shop. Ask their advice on which ones to buy.

5:2 Know-How

FINAL INSPIRATIONS

One of themes of this book has been community, so I asked members of the forum and Facebook group to sum up in a sentence or two what 5:2 means to them. Their answers are inspiring.

> 5:2 has given me freedom from the tyranny of diets, the tools to help me lose weight and keep it off, and the knowledge that I am doing something positive for my health now and in the future.

> **5:2 has been totally life-transforming for me. I was an overweight couch potato; now I'm a size 10 and run 5k three times a week.**

> It's the diet that's not a diet. You fit it round your life, you don't have to squeeze your life around it.

> **Weight loss is a bonus; it's all about physical and mental wellbeing for me.**

> 5:2 has finally given me an understanding of food, and respect for myself.

No mess, no fuss, just pounds away. . . Can't get better then that!

5:2 has given me CONFIDENCE! Not just losing weight, which is brilliant (I've lost 7kg [16 lbs] in two months) but it's given me a sense of control and a sense that I can actually face a challenge and cope.

I look forward to my two days a week, as I feel I am doing my body some good. This is a mind and health boost for me. Loving the way I feel and the way I look. And that hasn't happened in years.

It has stopped me from looking at foods in terms of good and bad.

5:2 marked the start of a new chapter in my life and opened the door to a new way of living. I have lost 10.5kg (23 lbs) in nine weeks. To be continued . . .

CHAPTER TEN

5:2 Menu Plans Made Easy

FOUR WEEKS OF FAST DAY MEAL-PLANNING MADE EASY

5:2 gives you so much freedom that it can be overwhelming – these meal plans are designed to help. Each week has one meal for women at around 500 calories, and one for men with 100 more – but they're just suggestions.

Planning your Fast Days really does increase your chances of success so do spend a little time in advance making sure you don't have to go shopping on the day.

Remember that not everything you eat has to be cooked from scratch, or come from a recipe in this book! Use the calorie counter on pages 338–347 to calculate counts for fruit or vegetable snacks, or side dishes of rice or couscous. And don't overlook simple options like beans on 1 slice wholemeal toast (200g of beans will be around 144, plus 92 for the toast) or chiller cabinet soups and low-calorie ready meals if you haven't had a chance to make your own.

Don't forget to allow for milk or almond milk if you take it in hot drinks.

If you're just getting started with 5:2, it's a very good idea to pre-plan a couple of very low-calorie snack options for emergencies. Pre-packed low-sugar jellies aren't quite the gourmet treat of our elderflower version, but they're typically under 10 calories and can be good for moments when you need something sweet, as are instant low-calorie hot chocolates, like Options, which are around 40 calories.

If you prefer something savoury, then ten pitted olives are around 45–50 calories, a Light Babybel is 40 or a low-calorie miso or cup-a-soups vary between 25–60 calories.

There are more tips and snack ideas on the forums or in *The 5:2 Diet Book*. The name of the game is flexibility – do whatever suits you best.

WEEK 1 (three meals a day)

Fast day 1: (for women: 490 calories)
Breakfast: Mushroom and Spinach Omelette Muffin *83 cals*
Lunch: Ruby Soup *82 cals*
Dinner: Crunchy Buttermilk Chicken with Balsamic
  Roasted Tomatoes and Courgettes *325 cals*

Fast day 2 (for men: 605 calories)
Breakfast: Berry Blast Smoothie made with almond milk and
  sesame seeds *171 cals*

Lunch: Panzanella Salad *152 cals*
Dinner: Lamb Kofta with Cucumber Salad and Minty Yoghurt Sauce *280 cals*

WEEK 2 (breakfast and dinner plus 1 snack)

Fast day 1: (for women: 493 calories)
Breakfast: Granola Square *148 cals*
Snack: Skinny Rarebit *96 cals*
Dinner: Basil and Lemon Salmon en Papillote with Roasted Fennel *136 cals* with 30g baby spinach salad and 1 teaspoon balsamic dressing *13 cals*

Fast day 2 (for men: 595 calories)
Breakfast: Speedy Baked Egg with Tomato and Ham *138 cals*
Snack: Tzatziki Dip with crudités – ½ red pepper, ½ medium cucumber chopped into dippers *60 cals*
Dinner: Spaghetti Bolognese *397 cals*

WEEK 3 (lunch and dinner)

Fast day 1: (for women: 504 calories)
Lunch: Chargrilled Vegetable Salad with Wholewheat Giant Couscous and Goat's Cheese *249 cals*
Dinner: Claire's Diet Coke Chicken *222 cals* plus Cauliflower Rice *16 cals* and 50g steamed baby sweetcorn/sugar snap pea mix *17 cals*

Fast day 2 (for men: 587 calories)
Lunch: Tuna Niçoise Wrap *298 cals* plus 1 kiwi fruit *42 cals*
Dinner: Sticky Indonesian Pork Stir-Fry *247 cals*

WEEK 4 (1 main meal)

Fast day 1: (Summer menu for women: 489 calories)
Main meal:
Gazpacho with croutons and garnish *110 cals*
Thai Prawn Skewers with Griddled Courgette, Pea and Mint
Salad *233 cals*
Strawberry and Basil Granita *146 cals*

Fast day 2 (Winter menu for men: 615 calories)
Main meal:
Spicy Chicken, Courgette, Basil and Orzo Soup *134 cals*
Skinny Chilli con Carne *246 cals* with Cauliflower Rice
16 cals
Banana Oaf Muffin *219 cals*

3

THE

5:2

TOOL KIT

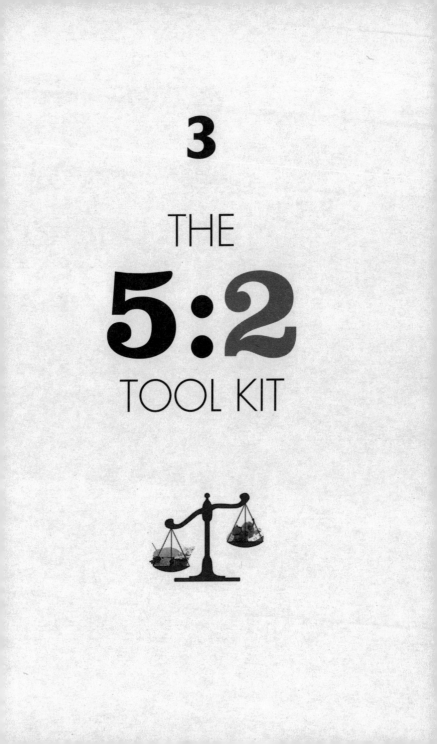

Recipes Listed by Calorie Count Per Serving:

The recipes are listed in alphabetical order, with two listings under different categories if there's a lower-calorie option.

Under 100

Asparagus, Mon Amour *66 cals*

Baba Ganoush Dip *74 cals*

Belinda's Raw Vegetable Salad with a Zingy, Spicy Dressing *88 cals*

Berry Fruit Compote *76 cals*

Cauliflower Rice *16 cals*

Courgette 'pasta' *34 cals*

Creamy Herb Dressing *5 cals per teaspoon*

Drinks including Chai, Mini-Mocha, Cosmopo-light-an, Nojito, all under *50 cals*

Elderflower Jellies with Blueberries, Mint and Raspberries (with sweetener) *39 cals*

Fruity Salsa *38 cals*

Garam Masala Spiced Mushrooms *71 cals*

Gazpacho *81 cals* (*or 110 cals with croutons and garnish*)

Gimlet cocktail *87 cals*

Jacqueline's Swamp Juice *98 cals*

Mushroom and Spinach Omelette Muffins *83 cals*

Mushroom Soup (without brandy and chestnuts) *48 cals*

Mushroom Stroganoff *70 cals*

Ruby Soup *82 cals*

Nutty Asian Dressing *17 cals per teaspoon*

Roasted Squash Hummus *94 cals*

Skinny Rarebit *95 cals*

Smoky Salsa *19 cals*

Strawberry and Basil Granita made with sweetener *56 cals*

Sweet and Sour Balsamic Dressing *5 cals per teaspoon*

The Only Tomato Sauce You'll Ever Need *30 cals (plus variations up to 40 cals)*

Tzatziki *36 cals*

Vietnamese Prawn Summer Rolls *84 cals per roll*

West Country dressing and Piquant Italian Dressing *26 cals per teaspoon*

Under 200

Asian Seared Beef with Rainbow Stir-Fry *186 cals*

Basil and Lemon Baked Salmon en Papillote with Roasted Fennel *171 cals*

Beef Pho *183 cals without noodles*

Berry Blast Smoothie *139–161 cals*

Brandied Mushroom and Chestnut Soup *143 cals*

Cinnamon and Vanilla Poached Pears *155 cals (129 cals without crème fraîche)*

Elderflower Jellies with Blueberries, Mint and Raspberries *102 cals*

Emma's Jaffa Cake Chocolate Mousse *152 cals*

Fast Day Trifle Treats *120–200 cals*

Granola Squares *148 cals*

Hearty Tuscan Bean Soup *136 cals (110 cals without ham)*

Kirsty's Butternut Squash and Sweet Potato soup *180 cals*

Lemon and Pork Meatballs *160 cals*

Panch Phoran Tomato and Red Lentil Soup *118 cals*

Panzanella *154 cals*

Skinny Mini Popeye Pies *199 cals*

Speedy Baked Egg with Tomato and Ham *138 cals*

Spicy Chicken, Courgette, Basil and Orzo Soup *134 cals*

Spring Vegetable and Pesto Minestrone *127 cals (106 cals without cheese)*

Strawberry and Mint Granita *146 cals*

Sweet Potato Falafel *189 cals without pitta*

Thai Green, Red, Yellow (or whatever colour you like) Curry *170 cals*

Trio of Twisted Waldorf Salads *125–176 cals*

Under 300

Avocado Wraps with Lettuce/Little Gem 'Open Sandwiches' *229 cals*

Banana Oat Muffins *219 cals*

Becca's Perfect Pizza *246 cals*

Beef Pho *260 cals*

Best Vegetarian Cottage Pie *272 cals*

Bottom-of-the-Fridge Frittata *200–300 cals*

Chargrilled Vegetable Salad with Wholewheat Giant Couscous and Goat's Cheese *249 cals*

Claire's Diet Coke Chicken *222 cals*

Greek Spring Lamb Stew *239 cals*

Huevos 'Fasteros' *230 cals*

Kate's Saag Paneer *220 cals*

Lamb Kofta with Cucumber Salad and Minty Yoghurt Sauce
  280 cals
Lizzie's Harira *284 cals*
Naughty Rarebit *228 cals*
One-Tray Baked Cod Provençal *247 cals*
Richard's Cosmo *224 cals*
Skinny Chilli con Carne *246 cals*
Smoked Chicken and Mango Salad *237 cals*
Spicy Mexican Bean Burgers without bun etc *244 cals*
Sticky Banana and Date Bread *185 cals*
Sticky Indonesian Pork Stir-Fry *247 cals*
Thai Prawn Skewers with Griddled Courgette, Pea and Mint
  Salad *233 cals*
Tuna Niçoise Wraps *298 cals*
Udon Noodle Miso Soup *226 cals*
Vanilla Granola *231 cals*
Vegetable Biryani *253 cals*
Warm Puy Lentil, Roasted Peppers and Spinach Salad with
  Basil Yoghurt Dressing *238 cals*

Under 400

Avocado Wraps with tortilla wraps *322 cals*
Chicken, Lemon and Olive Tagine *312 cals without couscous*
Crunchy Buttermilk Chicken with Balsamic Roasted
  Tomatoes and Courgettes *324 cals*
Fiona's Asian Chicken Lettuce Wraps *319 cals*
Jerk Chicken *316 cals without rice*
Lemon and Asparagus Risotto *308 cals*

Quinoa with Feta and Peas with Lemon, Honey and
   Hazelnut Dressing *309 cals (no avocado)*
Roasted Beetroot, Pecan and Goat's Cheese Salad with
   Watercress and Chicory *329 cals*
Seared Tuna Steak with Five-Bean Salad and Rocket Dressing
   379 cals
Skinny Chicken Kievs *378 cals*
Spaghetti Bolognese *397 cals (211 cals sauce only)*
Spicy Vietnamese Chicken Noodle Salad with Lime, Mint
   and Chilli Dressing *338 cals*
Sweet Potato Falafel Pockets *334 cals*

Under 500

Beef and Ale Stew *439 cals*
Chicken, Lemon and Olive Tagine *406 cals*
Coriander, Lime and Chilli Prawn Pasta *440 cals*
Grilled Mackerel with Roast Beetroot, Watercress and
   Horseradish and Balsamic Dressing *405 cals*
Hot Smoked Salmon and Watercress Linguini *464 cals*
Jerk Chicken with Coconut Rice and Pineapple Chilli Salsa
   481 cals
Lamb Kofta in Pitta Pockets with Feta, Cucumber Salad and
   Minty Yoghurt Sauce *443 cals*
Quinoa with Feta, Avocado and Peas with Lemon, Honey
   and Hazelnut Dressing *426 cals*
Spicy Mexican Bean Burgers with all the trimmings *458 cals*

Calorie Counter

Many of the ingredients in this book are listed below, with both calories per 100g/ml and also the calories in an average portion or serving. These are all actually Kilocalories (kcal on food labels) but most of us call these calories, so that's what we're using.

As I said in the introduction to Think Like a 5:2 Cook (see pages 36–38), calorie counting is an inexact science. We've offered averages for most produce based on a variety of sources. Where a range is shown, do check the labels on branded or packaged goods to compare. You're unlikely to go far off course with white wine vinegar, for example, but higher fat or calorie products could derail your Fast Day. Also see the note about herbs and spices in the same chapter (see page 39), and about the variability of homemade and shop-bought stock (see page 40).

We have checked recipes and calorie counts six times, but it is still possible that errors may have crept in: if you spot one, I apologise! But I hope you'll use this tool to keep you on track!

Food	Calories per 100g/ml	Average serving size	Calories per average portion
DAIRY			
Cheeses			
Brie	305	25g	76
Cheddar, full-fat mature	400	25g	100
Cheddar, reduced-fat	215–275	25g	54–69
Cheddar, slices, reduced-fat	240	25g slice	60

Food	Calories per 100g/ml	Average serving size	Calories per average portion
Feta, full-fat	360	15g	54
Feta-style, light salad cheese	180	15g	27
Fromage frais, fat-free	50	1 tablespoon	8
Goat's cheese	270–330	25g	68–83
Halloumi, reduced-fat	255	50g	128
Lancashire	370	25g	93
Parmesan	415	10g	42
Philadelphia Light	146–160	1 tablespoon	22–24
Quark	69	1 tablespoon	10
Ricotta	134	1 tablespoon	20

Milk and yoghurt/substitutes			
Almond milk	13	1 tablespoon	2
Coconut milk	233	1 tablespoon	35
Coconut milk, reduced-fat	73–210	1 tablespoon	11–32
Coconut (non-dairy) yoghurt	165	1 tablespoon	25
Cow's milk, semi-skimmed	49	1 tablespoon	7
Cow's milk, skimmed	35	1 tablespoon	5
Crème fraîche, half-fat	170	1 tablespoon	26
Greek yoghurt, fat-free	55	1 tablespoon	8
Greek yoghurt, full-fat	130	1 tablespoon	20
Soya milk, unsweetened	20–34	1 tablespoon	3–5

Food	Calories per 100g/ml	Average serving size	Calories per average portion
Eggs			
Egg, large		1 egg	100
Egg, medium		1 egg	78
Egg white		1 egg white	14
BREADS, GRAINS (GRAINS ALL GIVEN AS DRY WEIGHT) AND BAKING			
Baking powder	100	1 teaspoon	5
Barley couscous	340	25g	85
Basmati rice, brown	330	25g	83
Basmati rice, white	355	25g	89
Bread, white	220	1 slice from smaller loaf, 25g	55
Bread, wholemeal	220	1 slice from smaller loaf, 25g	55
Bulgar wheat	360	25g	90
Couscous	376	25g	94
Egg noodles	220–355	25g	55–89
Flour, white	335	1 teaspoon	17
Flour, wholewheat	310	1 teaspoon	16
Pasta, white	233–360	25g	58–90
Pasta, wholewheat	330	25g	83
Porridge oats/rolled oats	355	25g	89
Quinoa	365	25g	91
Tortilla, corn	270–340	1 tortilla wrap	117
Tortilla, white wheat	270–340	1 tortilla wrap	100–200

Food	Calories per 100g/ml	Average serving size	Calories per average portion
VEGETABLES AND SALADS			
Asparagus	27	4 spears	13
Aubergine	20	1 small (60g)	12
Avocado (varies according to variety)	156-190	Small–medium avocado (150-200g)	235–380
Baby sweetcorn and sugar snap pea mix	33	50g	17
Beetroot	43	1 medium beetroot	35
Bell pepper	30	1 medium red pepper	30
Broccoli	32	½ small head	32
Cabbage	26	½ head cabbage (130g)	34
Carrot	34	1 medium (100g)	34
Cauliflower	25	½ small head (130g)	32
Celeriac	29	½ celeriac (75g)	22
Celery	10	1 medium stick (60g)	6
Courgette	20	1 medium (170g)	34
Cucumber, with peel	14	½ medium cucumber	15
Edamame beans	130	50g	65
Fennel	31	½ medium fennel	31
Garlic	110	1 clove	4

Food	Calories per 100g/ml	Average serving size	Calories per average portion
Green beans	27	50g	14
Leeks, raw	22	1 medium (180g)	40
Lettuce	15	30g	5
Mushrooms, dried	250	5g	13
Mushrooms, fresh	13	100g	13
Mushrooms, portobello	26	1 portobello	18
Mushrooms, shiitake	25	50g	13
Onion, red or white	38	1 medium, peeled	38
Onion, spring	32	1 small	1–2
Pak choi	17	1 head	17
Peas, garden, frozen	70	30g	22.5
Peas, petit pois, frozen	50	30g	15
Potato, white	85	1 small potato, baked	139
Radish	13	3 medium	3
Rocket	24	Handful	2
Spinach	25	30g	8
Squash, e.g. butternut	40	50g	20
Sweetcorn	90	1 cob 1 tablespoon	120 14
Sweet potato, uncooked	90	1 small	90–120
Tomatoes, fresh	20	1 medium 1 cherry tomato	16 3–5
Tomatoes, chopped and tinned	18	400g tin	72
Watercress	26	Handful	3

Food	Calories per 100g/ml	Average serving size	Calories per average portion
FRUIT			
Apple, with skin	47–50	1 medium dessert	60–95
Apricots, dried	250	3 dried, ready-to-eat	16
Apricot, fresh	48	1	17
Banana	105	1 small	89
Blackberries	40	50g	20
Blueberries	57	50g	29
Cherries	60	10 cherries	50
Cranberries, dried	340	15g	51
Dates, Medjool	287	30g	86
Dried mixed fruit	200–290	10g	20–29
Goji, dried	300	15g	45
Grapes	60	10 grapes	34
Kiwi fruit	55	1 kiwi fruit	42
Lemon, whole	29	1 lemon	19
Lemon juice, bottled	50	1 teaspoon	2.5
Lime	30	1 lime	20
Mango	60	½ medium mango (100–150g)	60–90
Orange, whole	37	1 orange	70
Papaya	39	½ medium (150g)	60
Passion fruit, flesh and seeds	36	1 passion fruit	17
Peach	35	1 medium	51
Pear	40	1 medium	50–90

Food	Calories per 100g/ml	Average serving size	Calories per average portion
Pineapple	50	30 g	14
Pomegranate seeds	82	1 tablespoon	12
Raisins, seedless	300	1 tablespoon	42
Raspberries	38	50g	19
Rhubarb, stewed, no sugar	7	1 tablespoon	1.5
Strawberries	32	50g	16
Sultanas	300	1 tablespoon	42
Tangerine	35	1 tangerine	40
Watermelon	31	50g chunk	16
PROTEINS			
Baked beans Reduced sugar and salt	84 66	100g 100g	84 66
Beef, lean	177	100g	177
Beef, minced Beef, minced, extra-lean	209 120–180	100g 100g	209 120–180
Chicken breast, skinless	165	100g	165
Chickpeas, dried	320	25g	80
Chickpeas, tinned	108 (drained weight)	240g (drained weight)	260
Cod	96	150g fillet	144
Ham, sliced	84–92	1 wafer-thin slice	5–19
Ham, tinned	85–116	100g	85–116
Lamb, minced	208	100g	208
Mackerel, raw Mackerel, smoked	153 260	100g 100g	153 260
Parma ham	220	14g slice	31

Food	Calories per 100g/ml	Average serving size	Calories per average portion
Pork, lean	182	100g	182
Pork tenderloin	140	100g	140
Prawns, king	70–80	100g	70-80
Red lentils, dry	330	25g	82.5
Salmon, fillet	140–215	1 small fillet (70g)	100 (approx.)
Salmon, smoked	220	50g	110
Sea bass	160	100g	160
Tofu	85–185	100g	85–185
Tuna, fresh Tuna, tinned in brine	136 99	100g 100g	136 99
Turkey	155	100g	155
White beans, tinned	76	100g	76

Nuts and seeds			
Almonds, flaked, ground	630	15g	94.5
Almonds, whole, with skin	610	1 almond	7
Brazils	680	1 nut	20–24
Chestnuts, vacuum-packed	160	15g	24
Coconut, dried, flaked	635	15g	95
Hazelnuts	668	15g	100
Peanuts, unsalted	564	15g	85
Pecans	698	15g	105
Pine nuts	695	15g	104
Pistachios	594	1 nut	6

Food	Calories per 100g/ml	Average serving size	Calories per average portion
Poppy	556	1 teaspoon	28
Pumpkin seeds	582	1 teaspoon	29
Sunflower	612	1 teaspoon	30
Sesame	634	1 teaspoon	32
Walnuts	690	15g	104

Stocks			
Beef	5	500ml	25
Chicken	4	500ml	18–20
Vegetable	2.5	500ml	13
Marigold stock bouillon powder	240	1 teaspoon	12
Sweeteners			
Agave nectar	300–340	1 teaspoon	15–17
Chocolate, 70% dark	510–570	1 small square	30
Cocoa powder, unsweetened	345	1 teaspoon	5
Honey	300–340	1 teaspoon	20
Maple syrup	255–330	1 teaspoon	13–17
Sugar, white/brown	395–400	1 teaspoon	15
Truvia baking blend	250	1 teaspoon	10

Flavourings and sauces			
Branston pickle	109	1 tablespoon	16
Curry pastes	120–260	1 tablespoon	18–39
Ketchup	115	1 tablespoon	17
Mango chutney	200–280	1 tablespoon	30–42
Most ground and whole spices	100		5 per tsp; 0 per pinch

Food	Calories per 100g/ml	Average serving size	Calories per average portion
Most leafy fresh herbs	50		0 for a few leaves; 5 per handful/10g/ tablespoon, chopped
Olives, pitted, in brine	100–133	5 olives	25
Passata	30	1 tablespoon	5
Salsa	30–70	1 tablespoon	5–11
Soy sauce	35–50	1 teaspoon	2–2.5
Tomato chutney	130–160	1 tablespoon	19.5–24
Tomato purée	30–93	1 tablespoon	5–14
Worcestershire sauce	113	1 teaspoon	5
Vinegars and mustards			
Balsamic vinegar	54–107	1 tablespoon	5–20
Cider vinegar	18	1 tablespoon	2
Red/white wine vinegar	22	1 tablespoon	2–3
English mustard	175	1 teaspoon	9
Mustard powder	520	½ teaspoon	13
Dijon mustard	100–150	1 teaspoon	5–10
Wholegrain mustard	154	1 teaspoon	8

Drinks			
Ale	25–47	½ pint	71–133
Apple juice	36–49	125ml	45–61
Black coffee	0–2	1 cup	0–5
Black tea	0	1 cup	0
Cava/Champagne	76	125ml	95

Food	Calories per 100g/ml	Average serving size	Calories per average portion
Lager	29–43	½ pint	82–122
Orange juice	36–43	125ml	45–54
Stout	21–39	½ pint	60–111
Spirits, e.g. gin, vodka	222	25ml single measure	56
Wine, dry white	66	125ml	83
Wine, red	68	125ml	85

Fats			
All oils, e.g. coconut, olive, sesame	899	1 teaspoon	45
Butter	744	1 teaspoon	37
Butter, reduced-fat	377–570	1 teaspoon	19–29

Glossary

5:2, 6:1, 4:3   Different variations on fasting/calorie restriction. The second number is the number of Fast Days.

ADF   Alternate Daily Fasting – cutting down or eating nothing every other day.

Bit.ly   Nothing to do with fasting, but a very useful way of shortening long web links in the links section that follows. You can type these directly into your browser to find a recommended web page.

BMI   Body Mass Index – a simple height/weight calculation used to gauge whether someone's weight may be putting their health at risk.

BMR   Basal Metabolic Rate – what your body needs in calorie terms for basic survival, without any activity other than basic functions

DCR   Daily Calorie Requirement – an estimate of the number of calories you need that factors in your activity levels as well as age, height and weight. See also TDEE.

Fast	'Fast' usually means eating nothing (and, in some religions, not drinking anything either). However, 5:2 dieters use it as shorthand for days when they eat limited amounts.
Feast	Days when you eat normally. Also known as Feed Days, Free Days, Normal days or whatever you want to call them!
Harris Benedict formula	A formula for estimating how many calories you need for daily life. Used by most online calculators, though the Mifflin St Jeor is seen as more accurate (see below).
IF/ICR	Intermittent Fasting or Intermittent Calorie Restriction. The latter is the more accurate name for the 5:2 approach.
Kcal	Kilocalorie is the accurate name for what most people call 'calories'.
Mifflin St Jeor formula	The more accurate formula for estimating your daily calorie needs.
TDEE	Total Daily Energy Expenditure – another name for Daily Calorie Requirement.

BMI Chart

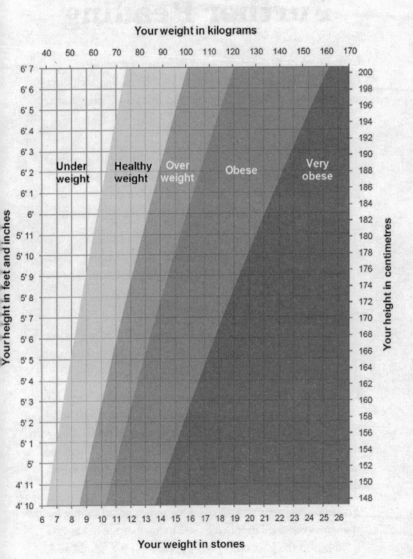

Your weight in kilograms

40 50 60 70 80 90 100 110 120 130 140 150 160 170

Your height in feet and inches

6' 7
6' 6
6' 5
6' 4
6' 3
6' 2
6' 1
6'
5' 11
5' 10
5' 9
5' 8
5' 7
5' 6
5' 5
5' 4
5' 3
5' 2
5' 1
5'
4' 11
4' 10

Your height in centimetres

200
198
196
194
192
190
188
186
184
182
180
178
176
174
172
170
168
166
164
162
160
158
156
154
152
150
148

Under weight

Healthy weight

Over weight

Obese

Very obese

6 7 8 9 10 11 12 13 14 15 16 17 18 19 20 21 22 23 24 25 26

Your weight in stones

Online Links and Further Reading

Our site, www.the5-2dietbook.com, features extensive information about this approach to healthy eating, including success stories and news. You can also contact me via the site.

Health and 5:2

These two digests/reviews of research (just type either of these shortened links directly into your browser address bar: bit.ly/113ykL3 and bit.ly/ShaV4h) give good overviews of intermittent calorie restriction and fasting and the effect on health.

For a comprehensive free list of links dealing with the science and research behind 5:2, go to www.the5-2dietbook.com/freebies

Forums and tools:

The forum at www.the5-2dietbook.com/forums is free to join and we'd love to see you there. Or come and join our Facebook group www.facebook.com/groups/the52diet

Donate Your Dinner is the 5:2 appeal. Many of us have chosen to donate the money we save on Fast Days (by skipping snacks or spending less on groceries, for example) to charities dealing with disadvantage and homelessness, including the UK's Foodbank network and Shelter. Find out more at www.justgiving.com/donateyourdinner

MyFitnessPal (myfitnesspal.com) has thousands of calorie listings, though as these are supplied by site users, they are not always reliable. On the plus side, it has a great app for Android and iPhone (free at the time of writing), which helps you track your weight, exercise and calorie consumption. It doesn't have a 'Fast Day' mode currently which means it may nag you to eat more on Fast Days and less on normal days so set it to 'maintenance mode' for normal days and only count to 5–600 on Fast Days.

You can calculate your TDEE and BMR on the same site or on www.fitnessfrog.com/calculators

More Recipes

The excellent BBC Good Food recipe site allows you to specify courses, ingredients, preparation time and calorie counts: www.bbcgoodfood.com

Jacqueline and Fiona, whose recipes feature in Chapter 1 and Chapter 6, contribute to this inspiring Pinterest board: pinterest.com/LavenderLovage/5-2-diet-recipes-for-fast-days

Further Reading

To learn more about my own 5:2 journey – and read the science and many more tips from 5:2 dieters – *The 5:2 Diet Book* is also published by Orion.

Acknowledgements

This book has been a labour of love – and a real group effort, bringing together ideas, knowledge and foodie enthusiasms of many people around the world.

First of all, I want to thank the members of the Facebook group and the 5:2 forum for the support, the stories and the generosity of spirit. It's so inspiring to hang out with you, and though the word 'community' is sometimes over-used, it really does feel like we've created a safe haven online.

Particular thanks to the talented cooks who have allowed me to print their stories and recipes: Simone Baker, Lizzie and Kevin Baker, Kirsty Badham, Belinda Berry, Becca Blake, Claire Cowking, Emma Hasson, Fiona Maclean and Jacqueline Meldrum.

Many thanks too for the brilliant team who volunteered to help me run the online community (4,000+ now in the Facebook group alone): Anita, Boo, Celia, Elaine, Ellie, Erika, Jo, Josie, Julie, Linda, Lolly, Megan, Natasha, Skids, Suzie, Tamara, Tracey, Victoria and Wai. You rock, guys and gals.

Recipe books usually take years to develop so turning this one round so quickly has meant some very long hours in some very hot kitchens. Thanks so much to culinary goddesses Anna Burges-Lumsden and Lisa Harrison for making the recipes work perfectly. To Cath Quinn for checking my nutritional know-how and to Pamela Brooks

354

for reading so carefully. And to the copy editor, Laura Herring, for a brilliant job.

Special thanks to the team at Orion, but especially to Jillian Young for pulling everything together in time for the scary deadlines against the odds!

And for 5:2 dedication, thanks to Peta, Sophie and Araminta for keeping me going in those moments when I did think the calorie count of half an avocado or a teaspoon or porridge oats would actually send me over the edge.

Special thanks to friends and family, and especially Rich, for putting up with me while my head has been full of DCR, BMR and serving sizes.

Lastly, thanks to *you* for buying this book.

If you have any comments or suggestions, you can get in touch via the 5:2 website, the 5-2dietbook.com or via my personal website for all my books, www.kate-harrison.com. I'd love to hear how you're making 5:2 work for you!

Kate x

Index

Badham, Kirsty 70–4
Baker, Kevin and Lizzie 102–7
Baker, Simone 299–304
Basal Metabolic Rate (BMR)
    15–16
Berry, Belinda 167–71
Blake, Becca 234–9
Body Mass Index (BMI) 23–4,
    351
budget tips 230–1

calorie counting 22, 26–7
    calculating limits 15–17
    calorie requirements 14
    individual foods 340–9
    individual recipes 335–9
    weighing ingredients 39–40
cold drinks 288–94
cooking methods 36–7
Cowking, Claire 134–9

Daily Calorie Requirement (DCR)
    14, 15, 16–17
diet principles 4
    calories required 15–17
    choice of foods 18–19
    exercise 20–1
    food on Feast Days 21–2
    hunger management 19–20
    timing of fast days 11–12, 13
    timing of meals 17–18, 23, 41
    weight loss targets 23–5

family meals 161–3
fats/oils 37–8
flavourings 127–31

Hasson, Emma 268–73
health benefits 3–4, 28–31, 38
holiday/celebration tips 264–5
hot drinks 283–8

kitchen equipment 95–9

lunchboxes 227–9

Maclean, Fiona 208–12
maintenance diet tips 295–6
Meldrum, Jacqueline 43–7
menu plans 326–9

pasta/potato alternatives 319–23

shirataki noodles 323
sprouting seeds 205
starvation mode 23
store cupboard ingredients 61–7
superfoods 195–201

veg boxes 202–4

waist/height ratio 24–5

zero noodles 323

Recipe Index

Asian dressing 119–20
Asian seared beef with rainbow
    stir-fry 119–20
asparagus 191–2, 256–7
avocado wraps 220–1

baba ganoush 242
baked egg with tomato and ham
    54–5
banana and date bread 225–6
banana oat muffins 48–9
basil and lemon salmon 151–2
basil yoghurt dressing 177–8
Becca's pizza 238–9
beef and ale stew 142–3
beef pho 91–2
beetroot, pecan and goat's cheese
    salad 185–6
Belinda's raw vegetable salad
    170–1
berry blast smoothie 224
berry compote 51
buttermilk chicken 149–50

chai 284–5
chargrilled vegetable salad 181–2
chicken, courgette, basil and orzo
    soup 85–6
chicken Kievs 157–8
chicken, lemon and olive tagine
    250–1
chilli con carne 125–6

cinnamon and vanilla pears 274–5
Claire's Diet Coke chicken 138–9
cod Provençal 155–6
coriander, lime and chilli prawn
    pasta 258–9
courgette 'pasta' 321–2
courgette, pea and mint salad
    254–5
creamy herb dressing 315

elderflower jellies 276–7
Emma's Jaffa cake chocolate
    mousse 271–3

Fiona's Asian chicken lettuce wraps
    211–13
frittata 243–5
fruity salsa 309

gazpacho 93–4
Gimlet cocktail 293
granola squares 222–3
grated vegetable salads 194–5
Greek lamb stew 252–3
Greek mezze 240–2

horseradish and balsamic dressing
    159–60
hot smoked salmon and watercress
    linguine 260
huevos 'fasteros' 59–60

Indonesian pork stir-fry 123–4

Jacqueline's swamp juice 46–7
jerk chicken with coconut rice
111–12

Kate's Cosmopo-light-an 292–3
Kate's mini mocha 287–9
Kate's saag paneer 113–15
Kirsty's butternut squash and
sweet potato 73–4

lamb kofta 117–18
lemon and asparagus risotto
256–7
lemon and pork meatballs 140–1
lemon, honey and hazelnut dressing 179–80
lime and herb dressing 174
lime, mint and chilli dressing
175–6
Lizzie's harira 106–7

mackerel with beetroot 159–60
Mexican bean burgers 261–3
mini Popeye pies 146–8
minty yoghurt sauce 118
mushroom and spinach omelette
muffins 52–3
mushroom rarebits 56–8
mushroom soup 78–80
mushroom stroganoff 246–7

Nojito cocktail 294
nutty Asian dressing 317

orange dressing 189–90

panch phoran tomato and red
lentil soup 87–8
panzanella 183–4
pineapple chilli salsa 111–12
piquant Italian dressing 314–15
poached eggs 193
Puy lentil salad 177–8

quinoa salad 179–80

raita 116
Richard's Cosmo 292
roasted tomatoes and courgettes
149–50
rocket dressing 172–3
ruby soup 75–7

Simone's cauliflower rice 303–4
smoked chicken and mango salad
174
smoky salsa 310-11
spaghetti Bolognese 144–5
spiced mushrooms 248–9
spring vegetable and pesto minestrone 83–4
squash hummus 240–1
stocks 316–18
strawberry and basil granita
278–9
sweet and sour balsamic dressing
313
sweet potato falafel 212–13

Thai curry 108–10
Thai prawn skewers 254–5
tomato sauces 140–1, 308–10
trifles 280–2
tuna Niçoise wraps 218–19
tuna steak with 5-bean salad
    172–3
Tuscan bean soup 81–2
tzatziki 241–2

udon noodle miso soup 89–90

vanilla granola pots 50–2
vegetable biryani 121–2

vegetarian cottage pie 153–4
Vietnamese chicken noodle
   salad 175–6
Vietnamese prawn rolls 216–17

Waldorf salads 187–90
West Country dressing 314

yoghurt dressing 188

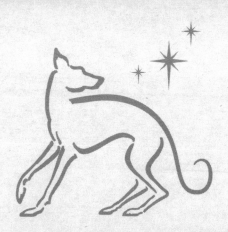